T0259056

Surgical Instruments

Guest Editor

KATHLEEN B. GABERSON, PhD, RN,
CNOR, CNE, ANEF

PERIOPERATIVE NURSING CLINICS

www.periopnursing.theclinics.com

Consulting Editor
NANCY GIRARD, PhD, RN, FAAN

March 2010 • Volume 5 • Number 1

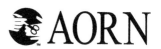

SAUNDERS an imprint of ELSEVIER, Inc.

W.B. SAUNDERS COMPANY

A Division of Elsevier Inc.

1600 John F. Kennedy Boulevard • Suite 1800 • Philadelphia, Pennsylvania 19103-2899

http://www.periopnursing.theclinics.com

PERIOPERATIVE NURSING CLINICS Volume 5, Number 1
March 2010 ISSN 1556-7931, ISBN-13: 978-1-4377-1857-7

Editor: Katie Hartner
Developmental Editor: Donald Mumford

Perioperative Nursing Clinics (ISSN 1556-7931) is published quarterly by Elsevier, 360 Park Avenue South, New York, NY 10010. Months of issue are March, June, September and December. Business and Editorial Offices: 1600 John F. Kennedy Blvd., Suite 1800, Philadelphia, PA 19103-2899. Customer Service Office: 11830 Westline Industrial Drive, St. Louis, MO 63146. Periodicals postage paid at New York, NY and at additional mailing offices. Subscription prices are $116.00 per year (domestic individuals), $213.00 per year (domestic institutions), $58.00 per year (domestic students/residents), $150 per year (international individuals), $245 per year (international institutions), and $62.00 per year (international students/residents). Foreign air speed delivery is included in all *Clinics* subscription prices. All prices are subject to change without notice. **POSTMASTER:** Send change of address to *Perioperative Nursing Clinics*, Customer Service (orders, claims, online, change of address): Elsevier Periodicals Customer Service, 11830 Westline Industrial Drive, St. Louis, MO 63146. Tel: 1-800-654-2452 (U.S. and Canada). Fax: 314-523-5170. E-mail: journalscustomerservice-usa@elsevier.com (for print support); journalsonlinesupport-usa@elsevier.com (for online support).

Reprints. For copies of 100 or more, of articles in this publication, please contact the Commercial Rights Department, Elsevier Inc., 360 Park Avenue South, New York, NY 10010-1710; phone: (+1) 212-633-3813; fax: (+1) 212-462-1935; e-mail: reprints@elsevier.com.

Contributors

CONSULTING EDITOR

NANCY GIRARD, PhD, RN, FAAN
Consultant, Boerne; Clinical Associate Professor, Acute Nursing Care Department, University of Texas Health Science Center, San Antonio, Texas

GUEST EDITOR

KATHLEEN B. GABERSON, PhD, RN, CNOR, CNE, ANEF
Nursing Education Consultant, OWK Consulting, Pittsburgh, Pennsylvania

AUTHORS

KATHLEEN B. GABERSON, PhD, RN, CNOR, CNE, ANEF
Nursing Education Consultant, OWK Consulting, Pittsburgh, Pennsylvania

THEODORE HAINES, MD, MSc
Associate Professor, Department of Clinical Epidemiology and Biostatistics, Faculty of Health Sciences, Health Sciences Centre, McMaster University, Hamilton, Ontario, Canada

CYNTHIA K. HALVORSON, RN, MSN, CNOR
Perioperative Clinical Educator and Consultant, Maur, Switzerland

MARY GRACE HENSELL, RN, BSN, CNOR
OR Manager, Allegheny General Hospital, Pittsburgh, Pennsylvania

PATRICIA ANN HERCULES, RN, MS
Missouri City; Director, System Clinical Education, Memorial Hermann Healthcare System, Houston, Texas

AMY L. KENNEDY, RN, MSN, CNOR
Director, Program of Surgical Technology; Professor of Surgical Technology, Harrisburg Area Community College, Harrisburg, Pennsylvania

LINDA E. SABIN, RNC, PhD
Professor of Nursing, School of Nursing, University of Louisiana at Monroe, Monroe, Louisiana; Ridgeland, Mississippi

RAMON SHABAN, BSc(Med), BN, PGDipPH&TM, GCertInfCon, DipAppSc(Amb), MCHlth(Hons), MEd, RN, EMT-P, IPN, CICP, FRCNA
Research Centre for Clinical and Community Practice Innovation, Griffith Institute for Health and Medical Research, Griffith University and Princess Alexandra Hospital, Brisbane, Australia

MICHAEL SINNOTT, MBBS, FACEM, FRACP
Senior Staff Specialist, Department of Emergency Medicine, Princess Alexandra Hospital, Woolloongabba, Queensland, Australia

STEPHANIE SMITH STANFIELD, RN, BSN, CNOR
North Brownsville Surgery Center, Brownsville, Texas

BERNADETTE STRINGER, PhD
Project Program Manager, Occupational Health and Safety Agency for Healthcare in BC (OHSAH), Vancouver; Adjunct Professor, Faculty of Health Sciences, Simon Fraser University, Burnaby, British Columbia, Canada

Contents

Preface: The Tools of the Trade   ix

Kathleen B. Gaberson

**From Fingers to Miniaturization and Robots: An Overview of the History
of Surgical Instrumentation**   1

Linda E. Sabin

> This retrospective historical analysis examines the history of surgical in-
> struments in relation to the development of surgery as a discipline and sci-
> ence. Nursing implications are included for readers dedicated to research
> for the improvement in patient outcomes. A key to searching for a contem-
> porary answer to a problem is found best by examining what has hap-
> pened in the past.

Instrument Readiness: A Patient Safety Issue   15

Patricia Ann Hercules

> Operating room instrument and equipment readiness and availability are
> necessary to safeguard patient care. Using available data and real-life
> stories, this article defines, gives an historical overview, and outlines the
> existing professional standards on this issue. It elaborates on contributing
> factors such as availability, substitutions, stress, and distractions. It con-
> cludes that the health care profession should take a closer look at this
> as a patient safety issue.

Review of Best Practices and Literature on Instrument Counts   27

Cynthia K. Halvorson

> With a heightened emphasis on patient safety and a lowered tolerance for
> the occurrence of "never events" there is a need for improved practices.
> Evidence-based knowledge bridges this gap by providing direction for
> best practices that ensure consistent and sustained safe patient care
> and optimal outcomes. Perioperative nursing has a long-standing and
> well-respected position of advocating for safe patient care. With intimate
> knowledge of the counting process, perioperative nurses, as key stake-
> holders in the multidisciplinary approach, must contribute to the body of
> evidence regarding best practices for effective surgical counts.

The Hands-Free Technique: An Effective and Easily Implemented Work Practice   45

Bernadette Stringer and Theodore Haines

> The hands-free technique, whereby no two people touch the same sharp
> item simultaneously during surgery, is an effective work practice recom-
> mended to reduce the risk of blood-borne exposure. This technique can
> be implemented using receptacles, tables, or the surgical field. Compli-
> ance with the technique can be increased using a newly developed
> video/DVD available for viewing on the Internet.

"Scalpel Safety," not "Safety Scalpel": A New Paradigm in Staff Safety   **59**

Michael Sinnott and Ramon Shaban

> Scalpel injuries account for between 7% and 12% of all sharps injuries. Efforts to increase the awareness of potential hazards of sharps injuries and related prevention efforts began in the early 1980s. Research shows convincingly that a single-handed scalpel blade remover combined with a hands-free passing technique (HFPT) is a safe alternative choice to the safety scalpel. The concept of "scalpel safety" is based on providing nurses the freedom of choice to select the best safety device for their individual needs on a case-by-case basis. Team members can now choose between a safety scalpel and a single-handed scalpel blade remover combined with a HFPT to achieve the correct balance between patient safety and staff safety.

Instrumentation for Robotic Surgery   **69**

Mary Grace Hensell

> Robotic surgery is performed with a computerized system that interacts with the surgical field by means of a mechanical arm or arms. This article discusses the components of the system and the appropriate instrumentation for robotic surgery. Because of a unique feature of the robot arm drapes, they are considered part of the instrumentation, with economic implications. The proper use and care of robotic instruments is also discussed.

Teaching Surgical Instrumentation: Innovative Techniques   **83**

Amy L. Kennedy and Kathleen B. Gaberson

> Introducing surgical instrumentation to the novice perioperative nurse, nursing student, or surgical technology student is challenging and rewarding. This article explores effective teaching approaches. It reviews three learning domains, selected learning and teaching principles, and provides guidance for selecting appropriate learning activities. Finally, it suggests evaluation strategies to assess that learning.

Surgical Instruments: A Laughing Matter?   **89**

Stephanie Smith Stanfield

> Among the sources of humor in the operating room are anecdotes about the names or functions of surgical instruments or equipment. This article presents a collection of such jokes and stories, arranged in various categories, contributed by perioperative nurses and other members of the surgical team.

Index   **95**

FORTHCOMING ISSUES

June 2010
Radiology
Kathleen Gross, MSN, RN, BVC, CRN,
Guest Editor

September 2010
Sterilization and Disinfection
Terri Goodman-Kent, PhD, RN, CNOR,
Guest Editor

December 2010
Update: Infection Control
George Allen, RN, PhD, CNOR, CIC,
Guest Editor

RECENT ISSUES

December 2009
Pain, Analgesia and Anesthesia
Valerie Girard-Powell, RN, *Guest Editor*

September 2009
Research
Robin D. Froman, RN, PhD, FAAN,
Guest Editor

June 2009
Education
Jane C. Rothrock, DNSc, RN, CNOR, FAAN,
Guest Editor

THE CLINICS ARE NOW AVAILABLE ONLINE!

Access your subscription at:
www.theclinics.com

Preface: The Tools of the Trade

People have used tools since the Stone Age. The first stone, wood, and bone tools undoubtedly were used for tasks necessary to sustain life—killing predator animals and later hunting animals for food, removing animal skins and joining pieces together to use for clothing and shelter, cutting pieces of flesh, and grinding grains. Once tools were developed for these purposes, ancient peoples probably adapted them for similar uses, including cutting the human body in an attempt to relieve pain and heal illness. Finally, tools were designed specifically for such surgical uses, and eventually the surgical instruments of the modern age were developed. As surgical practice and techniques continue to evolve, new surgical instruments are developed and existing instruments are modified for new uses. With an ever-increasing array of surgical instruments in various materials, sizes, shapes, and technologies, one may take these tools of the trade for granted as they are used to treat disease, correct deformities, restore function, and relieve pain. But as more instrument options become available, one needs to recognize their important role in improving patient and staff safety and reducing operative time.

This issue on surgical instruments includes articles with various perspectives that may stimulate renewed appreciation for the advances in technology that make sophisticated, complex surgical techniques possible. At the same time, one needs to recognize some inherent risks associated with the use of surgical instruments, examine evidence that supports or refutes some traditional handling techniques, and learn new ways of handling and caring for instruments so that they may be used effectively and safely.

In the first article, Dr Linda Sabin, a nurse historian, reveals a fascinating history of surgical instrumentation, starting with the use of our own body parts—mouths, hands, and fingers—as implements for removing foreign bodies, relieving pain, or incising and draining an abscess. This historical analysis provides support for the concept that all surgical instruments function as extensions of these original tools. She also supplies documentation that the function of surgical instruments evolved to support changes in the practice of surgery.

Next, Patricia Hercules presents a compelling argument that instrument readiness is a best-practice standard for safe perioperative patient care. Her article, "Instrument Readiness: A Patient Safety Issue," proposes that the safety of patients undergoing surgical intervention depends on verification that surgical instruments are immediately available, functional, sterile, and ready for use when needed.

Cynthia Halvorson's article, "Review of Best Practices and Literature on Instrument Counts," identifies and reviews extant research evidence supporting best practices for surgical instrument counts and discusses implications and recommendations for preventing adverse events related to incorrect counts. Because incidents of retained foreign bodies during surgery persist despite widespread use of manual count protocols, they now are classified as "never events" and reportable sentinel events. Evidence-based knowledge provides direction for developing and implementing effective protocols for reporting and reconciling instrument count discrepancies.

Although many surgical team members may regard percutaneous injuries during surgery as an inevitable occupational hazard, Dr Bernadette Stringer and Dr Theodore

Perioperative Nursing Clinics 5 (2010) ix–x
doi:10.1016/j.cpen.2009.12.004

Haines advocate for the consistent use of hands-free methods of passing instruments to prevent such injuries. They review the evidence on the effectiveness of this work practice as a safety measure to decrease bloodborne exposure risk from percutaneous injury. They also discuss an effective method of educating surgical team members to increase compliance with this technique.

In an article also related to the prevention of injuries from scalpels and other sharps, Dr Michael Sinnott and Ramon Shaban call for an emphasis on scalpel safety rather than reliance on use of scalpels with active safety features. They present evidence that the use of so-called safety scalpels does not in fact reduce risk of scalpel injuries to surgeons, perioperative nurses, and scrub technologists, and they call for a new paradigm of scalpel safety involving the choice of scalpel with active safety features or a single-handed scalpel blade remover combined with hands-free passing technique. They propose that this choice should be made on a case-by-case basis and should consider both the patient and staff member safety.

In her article, "Instrumentation for Robotic Surgery," Mary Grace Hensell uses her experience with robotic surgical systems to write about the challenges of using and caring for robotic surgery instruments. She explains the components of robotic systems and emphasizes the need to consider drapes for the robotic instrument arms as instrument components. She offers helpful suggestions for caring for robotic instruments and provides lists of basic robotic instrument sets for various surgical procedures.

Amy Kennedy's article, "Teaching Surgical Instrumentation: Innovative Techniques," provides guidance for educators who must introduce surgical instruments to the novice perioperative nurse, nursing student, or surgical technology student. We explain how knowledge of the three domains of learning is important for designing instruction for learners, and emphasizes that learning objectives should be chosen carefully to match the level at which learners will be expected to demonstrate the desired learning outcomes. Offering examples from her experience as professor and director of a surgical technology program, she recommends teaching techniques that effectively introduce and sequence information and skill practice related to use and handling of surgical instruments.

The final article is a collection of jokes and humorous stories related to surgical instruments, compiled and organized by Stephanie Stanfield. These jokes, anecdotes, and funny stories were submitted by perioperative nurses and other surgical team members in response to a request posted on the Association of Operating Room Nurses e-Chapter Web site. Sharing such jokes and stories has long been part of the culture of the perioperative environment, helping us to build camaraderie, relieve stress, and make work more enjoyable.

These articles provide a range of perspectives on the past, present, and potential future of the use and care of surgical instruments in perioperative nursing practice. May we never again take for granted these tools of the trade, but instead, strive to use them in ways that produce optimum patient outcomes and promote safety for surgical staff members as well as patients.

Kathleen B. Gaberson, PhD, RN, CNOR, CNE, ANEF
OWK Consulting
213 Sharon Drive
Pittsburgh, PA 15221, USA

E-mail address:
kathygaberson@verizon.net

From Fingers to Miniaturization and Robots: An Overview of the History of Surgical Instrumentation

Linda E. Sabin, RNC, PhD[a,b,*]

KEYWORDS

• History • Surgical instruments • Surgical nursing

Surgery as a practice has ancient roots beginning with primitive attempts to help the sick by opening the body, piercing it, or changing it in some way in an attempt to help a person in need. Although this ancient craft has endured to modern times, it is important for nurses to remember that the practice of surgery as it is known today only has been a respected scientific discipline for a little over 150 years. In addition, like nurses, surgeons suffered some of the same frustrations in gaining full recognition for their contribution to medicine because of long periods of time when their practice did not progress.[1(p477)]

Nurses need to appreciate how surgical instruments were developed in relation to the history of surgery to anticipate what is likely to happen in the future. Kirkup noted that the dramatic changes in surgery and instrumentation were related directly to the development of anesthesia, antisepsis, asepsis, and other scientific advances, The long periods of slow advancement in the field, however, did provide the time to solve issues related to anatomy and other basics that allowed 19th century surgeons to take advantage of the allied developments. A key concept in understanding this history is to recognize that all surgical instruments function as extensions of the original tools that came from the human body: mouths, hands, and fingers.[2(ppxi, 42–3)] It is also important to recognize that the function of the instruments evolved with the practice of the art of surgery. It is impossible to separate the story of the tools surgeons use from the human saga that stimulated the need for surgery.

[a] School of Nursing, University of Louisiana at Monroe, 700 University Avenue, Monroe, LA 71209, USA
[b] 503 Charmant Place, Ridgeland, MS 39157, USA
* School of Nursing, University of Louisiana at Monroe, 700 University Avenue, Monroe, LA 71209.
E-mail address: Sabin@ulm.edu

Perioperative Nursing Clinics 5 (2010) 1–13
doi:10.1016/j.cpen.2009.11.005
1556-7931/10/$ – see front matter © 2010 Elsevier Inc. All rights reserved.

ANCIENT SOCIETIES

As noted previously, the earliest instruments for surgery were mouths, hands, and fingers. Fingers are capable of probing, manipulating, and retracting, and fingernails were used for cutting and scraping. Wrists and hands are capable of twisting, pounding, and pulling on body parts. Mouths can be used to suck out perceived poison or blood.[2(pp42–3)] One can picture the plight of primitive people using what they had to remove foreign objects, attempt to break a boil or abscess, or treat illnesses that caused pain and fevers. Before tools, bodies were all they had available. These first patients experienced all of the risks of surgery that remained problems until the 19th century AD: pain, risk of hemorrhage, and risk of infection. Although there is evidence that primitive people attempted to relieve pain by such means as drugs, alcoholic drinks, acupuncture, and mind-altering herbs, pain never was banished. There is also evidence that hemorrhage was recognized early as a problem and was treated with tourniquets, pressure, and cautery. When the history of surgical outcomes is examined, it is a tribute to human resilience that people ever survived major surgery prior to the modern era.[3(p38)]

As people evolved, they developed crude tools made of animal bone, antlers, horns, and stone, and began to use them to cut the human body and treat illness. Tools probably were developed for other daily activities and were put into use when a surgical need arose. The practice of using tools designed for a purpose unrelated to human surgery procedures would continue until modern times. Some of the earliest tools that have survived in physical form or in artistic images were knives or cutting blades, saws, scissors, tweezers, clamps, and crude drills. One of the earliest metals used was copper. Organic materials also were used such as shells to cut flesh and shark teeth to use as lancets and scarifiers. Canals from long animal bones and long hollow plant stems were used as conduits. Kirkup classified the major types of tools in terms of structure and form: probes, needles, spring forceps, catheters, scissors, clamps, retractors, and those instruments that have mixed forms.[2(pp80–2)]

There is considerable evidence from ancient writings, art drawings, and physical remains that one of the earliest surgical procedures practiced throughout human societies was trephination. The procedure consisted of drilling or cutting of holes in the skull to heal illness. Primitive healers performed trephination with the aid of knives, lancets, and other sharp objects. Evidence indicates that this surgery was performed to relieve illnesses such as headaches and epilepsy. Researchers have found reports and skulls verifying the practice in such widely separated regions as Peru and Egypt. Early alloyed metals and organic materials were used to fashion knives and hand-operated drilling tools to open bones in the head. One study examined trephined skulls from primitive Peruvian tribes and noted that 70% of the skulls showed evidence of healing, indicating that patients had survived.[2(p5),4(p8)]

Ancient Egyptian surgery progressed to the level of specialties, with each group of doctors responsible for a part of the body. For example, the physician in charge of the intestines would provide enemas and surface treatments, and the physician in charge of the head would do the trephining. An ancient (1500 BC) papyrus discovered in the 19th century describes surgical cases and strategies used, such as the patient with a "tumor and abscess." This disorder was treated with a "firedrill," which was a firestick used for kindling a wood fire in this period. The Egyptian surgeon had a hot point to probe an abscess.[3(p98),5(p17),6(p26)]

Hippocrates (400 BC) did not differentiate between physicians and surgeons, but wrote about a great variety of human disorders and their treatment. He wrote more about surgery than any other topic. Hippocrates recognized the four major elements believed to make up the body that were accepted in his era: water, earth, fire, and air. These elements had corresponding bodily characteristics: wet, dry, hot, and cold. The characteristics led to the theory of humors related to the fluids observed in the human body: blood, yellow bile, black bile, and phlegm. Many of the early surgical treatments were aimed at either enhancing or reducing those humors that were considered the cause of illness when they were out of balance. Surgical instruments described by Hippocrates were bronze or copper and of various natural materials such as animal horn.[2(p9),3(pp210-7),5(pp39-41)]

Many of his writings were about war wounds and care of broken bones including the use of iron rods. According to Hippocrates, war and surgery would always be linked because of the inevitable wounds that followed human conflict. His surgical writings also addressed more common problems such as anal fistula and included some interesting surgical equipment. The treatment recommended for the fistula was to introduce a ball of animal horn into the rectum and leave it there unless the patient needed to pass a stool.[2(p79)] He taught that observation was of prime importance in determining what the patient needs were. He also was a visionary who taught that diseases had specific causes, with many problems coming from the natural world, and that recovery could be assisted with surgery and medicine.[2(p79)] It is noteworthy that in Hippocrates' time, women were never accepted as either surgeons or nurses, and the only persons allowed to work with instruments in surgery besides the male surgeons were their apprentices. These assistants also gave the bedside care.[7(pp54-5)]

Galen (130 to 200 AD) followed Hippocratic ideas but redefined some of the earlier teachings and added to both the elemental and humoral theories. He focused on theological explanations related to disease and stressed his expanded views of humoral theory of illness. He also believed in observation of the patient and the use of medicine and surgical procedures to treat humoral imbalances. The primary surgical treatments used in the Galenic approach were bleeding, cupping, blistering, purging, and counterirritation. All of these painful processes were aimed at relieving excess humors believed to cause disease. Inflammation also was believed to cleanse the body of bad humors, so counterirritation could include scratching or scarifying the skin to cause reddening or small areas of bleeding. Nurses need to remember that these strategies were still in use in the United States well into the 19th century and often were employed as a defense against communicable fevers. Nurses at the bedside heated the tools for blistering or hot cups for the counterirritation. They also cleaned up after the bleeding procedures. In times of epidemic, a physician might have many calls to make, and it was up to those caring for the patient to follow the doctor with care and comfort, as well as cleaning up from whatever was performed while the doctor moved on to the next case. This approach to medicine and surgery was not challenged for over 1500 years after its development.[3(pp251-9),8(pp5,10)]

THE DARK PERIOD IN SURGICAL HISTORY

Following the advances of ancient civilizations and the Greeks, there was a long period of history when little surgery was performed in the Western world outside of a few university surgical centers such as Salerno (Italy) and Paris (France). Much of the surgical skill and practice was lost in the Middle Ages because of the dominance of the Catholic Church, which taught the primacy of the Holy Spirit to intercede in illness and forbade the educated monks and priests from spilling blood. Only the simplest of procedures related to Galenic theory were used in this period. Monks had maintained much of the practical medical knowledge after the fall of Rome but were limited by Papal edicts over time, and by the 12th and 13th centuries they had to send barbers or servants out into the community to perform bleeding, extraction of teeth, and other treatments. This led to the advent of barber surgeons.[1(p477)]

The movement of surgery out of the monasteries and into the universities lowered the public esteem for the surgeons and surgery. Attempts were made to improve the field with guilds and apprentice systems that survived to the 19th century, but prior to painless, germ-free surgery, the surgeons were tolerated as an inferior necessity when compared with other physicians. This situation did little to stimulate innovation or development in the field of surgical instrumentation. The state of surgery in the Middle Ages, even for the master surgeons in the universities, became brutal and one shunned by all but the most desperate. Nutting and Dock described the painful and pitiful state of surgery for the patient who had to experience surgery by being held down to a table, cut with a red hot knife, and then having the wound sealed with hot tar to prevent hemmorrhage.[1(pp478)]

Poor people without access to surgical tools returned to earlier periods and used fingernails and crude animal bone instruments. For example, midwives in this period used a long protected fingernail, grown just for this purpose, to cut the infant's frenulum at birth to prevent the problem of being tongue-tied. Animal teeth were used to break skin to promote bleeding. The tools used by these surgeons were often made of iron and were crude and clumsy. The types of tools included knives, probes, scissors, saws, needles, lithotomy sounds for kidney stones, and catheter sounds for bladder stones. These tools were made of metal and organic materials such as leather.[2(pp3,53)]

Innovation did continue in at least one area of practice: stone cutting. People had suffered from kidney and bladder stones since prehistoric times. Hippocrates recognized the need for specialists in this field. The process of lithotomy was practiced with increasing sophistication using various tools. Although the classic perineal approach to bladder stone removal had required simply a knife and scissors, innovators in the Middle Ages and early Renaissance began the practice of using fluted probes and special dilators to gain access to the bladder. By the late 18th century, surgeons had developed the suprapubic lithotomy to remove bladder stones.[7(pp146–7)]

WAR SURGERY IN THE MIDDLE AGES

A major change in the needs of soldiers in wartime took place in the 14th century. Until that time, war wounds resulted from battles with knives, swords, spears, arrows, and blunt instruments. The invention of gunpowder changed the injuries to gross tissue destruction and deep penetrating wounds with small wound tracts that allowed for infection with anaerobic microbes. This era led to the period of amputation as the primary surgical procedure in wartime. Surgeons confronted with multiple injuries abandoned removal of projectiles in the deeper organs because of the inevitable sepsis and death. Amputation was quicker, and more men survived. Most of those injured in the head or trunk developed serious infections; this stimulated the use of heat-based treatments such as boiling oil poured into deep wounds and more probe-shaped cautery to seal wounds.[9(pp127–8)]

Late in the Middle Ages, there was growing interest in anatomy in the medical community, and eventually dissection was begun, again in spite of Church objections. Interestingly, it would be this interest in the body that would reignite a brief resurgence of interest in surgery. Versalius (1514 to 1564) was a physician who advanced human understanding of anatomy with a classic work that detailed knowledge of the human body previously unknown to the medical world. He provided surgeons with information about body structures not previously studied and stimulated interest in corrective surgery. His work eventually would impact human understanding of anatomy and would lay a foundation for the rapid growth of surgical technique and instrument development in the 19th century. He was also a visionary and pioneer in surgical instrumentation. He developed a safe procedure for tracheotomy and created the instruments to maintain an airway and reinflate lungs, and demonstrated the process on pigs.[10] Unfortunately, in his era of the early 16th century, the theories of Galen conflicted with many of his insights and theories. Thus surgical practice lagged behind the theory because of the resistance of the medical profession to abandon Galen's precepts.[3(p416),8(p11)]

In this same period, Paré demonstrated that war wounds suffered by the French army would heal just as well without being treated with boiling oil or red-hot cautery to stop bleeding. He demonstrated the value of ligating arteries and preventing hemorrhage without the additional pain and suffering following the amputation of a limb. After the hemorrhage was controlled, he used a dressing of turpentine, rose oil, and egg yolk. Nutting and Dock credited his humane and gentle approach to patients as an example of nursing practice in the field of battle. His unwillingness to follow tradition allowed him to change the direction of wound care. He also created many innovative surgical instruments including fine tools for removing cataracts. His gentler, safer approach to surgery affected practice long after his era.[1(pp480–6),3(p381),9(p129),11(p4)]

15TH TO 19TH CENTURIES

As the Middle Ages began to give way to the Renaissance, there was a shift in practice toward specialization in surgery, and with the specialization came an interest in special tools for each area (eg, development and refinement of obstetric forceps and specialized stone-cutting tools). During this period, in addition to metal tools, instruments made of organic materials were common, especially in rural or poor regions where expensive equipment was rare. Animal horns were used for cupping, and beeswax tapers were used as probes and as surgical bougies to investigate urethral strictures. The wax would soften at body temperature to promote passage. Wax also was used to stop bleeding from the bone.[2(pp13,80),12(pp13–5)]

Little progress would be made in the field of surgery for another long period of time because of the lack of adjuncts now taken for granted such as anesthesia and asepsis. Most of the innovations and surgical manuals were developed between the 15th and 19th centuries by surgeons after war experiences in the battlefield or on the war ships of the day. During this period, amputation became the most common surgery because of the failure to successfully treat penetrating deep tissue wounds.[2(pp11–2)]

As late as the early 19th century, surgical care was still a dismal last resort for only the most desperate or war wounded. Dock and Stewart noted, "Surgery was in a worse state than it had been in the later Middle Ages and had a higher death rate… ." They noted that the techniques of Paré that heated instruments between patients and used alcohol to disinfect had helped in the past. But the early Victorians had depended on heavy poultices to promote pus that was believed to help repair tissues.[13(p115)] Nurses in surgical settings spent much of their time changing dressings and sitting with septic patients with fatal infections. In this era before the understanding of germ theory or anesthesia, nursing was a dangerous and disagreeable profession. This was the era that Nightingale encountered when she entered the Deaconess Institute at Kaiserswerth, Germany, in the 1850s. This also may have accounted for her life-long devotion to cleanliness as a protection against disease and infection after surgery. Today it is hard to envision the image of a surgeon wearing a blood-stained dirty apron and using instruments on one patient after another without thoroughly cleaning them, but it was a common practice in this period.[8(p34),14(pp141–54)]

ANESTHESIA

The year 1842 often is listed as a turning point in the history of surgery, because this was the time when anesthesia was introduced to make surgery painless. Long used sulfuric ether to perform painless surgery on three patients, but he did not report his experience initially. Two years later, Wells used nitrous oxide to remove teeth. He did report his findings. Although ether, chloroform, and nitrous oxide gas had been discovered in the 1830s, the medical value was not confirmed until the 1840s. The discovery of anesthesia ended a long period of what has been described as heroic surgery, when surgeons had to be quick and ambidextrous and were limited in the scope of what could be done for patients. There was such a need to hurry, because the patients had only analgesia and were still conscious. Surgeons based their reputations on daring, speed, and strength to complete procedures in record time to minimize suffering.[3(pp528–30),15,16(p7),17(p557)] Before the development of anesthesia, surgeons were limited severely in the scope and complexity of what they could achieve with a conscious patient. This also limited the demand for improved surgical instruments, because few complex time-consuming procedures were possible.[16(p8)]

AMERICAN EXPERIENCE IN THE 18TH AND EARLY 19TH CENTURIES

In the United States, physicians had to play the roles of physician, surgeon, and dentist from the colonial period and to the mid-19th century except in a few northeastern cities where pioneer medical centers were established. This meant that any physician had to be ready to do basic surgery related to the Galenic theory of humors (blistering, cupping, scarification, and bleeding). Physicians also had to pull teeth and provide dental care when it was needed. Specialization was still generations away for most physicians in the small communities in this country. This meant that each practitioner had to have a collection of medical equipment and surgical instruments, called the armamentarium by the manufacturers.[2(pp78–9),16(pp1–2),18(pp50,64)] The typical tools used by these physicians included knives; lancets; needles; clamps or pliers for tooth removal; amputation equipment such as tourniquet, saw, and ligatures; and in some cases obstetric equipment such as forceps. The metal tools were heavy (made of iron, brass, and carbon) and were finely crafted. The edges and borders of these tools were softened with organic materials such as leather or calf skin. Forceps might be lined with leather to increase friction and grasping ability.[2(pp78–9),16(pp1–2)]

SURGERY AFTER ANESTHESIA AND NEW INSTRUMENT DEVELOPMENT

The coming of anesthesia opened a new era of conservative surgery where the surgeon could move more slowly and preserve adjacent tissues, work deeper in the body, and use skill as well as speed to accomplish the task. Once surgeons were able to slow their actions and study the operative site with greater accuracy, there was the beginning movement away from the Galenic humors theory to a more organ-specific approach to the study of pathology.[2(pp78–9),16(pp1–2)] There was great interest in expanding surgical options for a new set of human ills after the development of painless surgery, and with this expansion came the growth of specialties in the urban centers of the country. This stimulated a demand for new instruments to provide the procedures needed. Specialties such as ophthalmology and urology required specialized equipment never considered prior to painless surgery. This expansion was prior to the discovery of the germ theory, and materials used in the manufacture of instruments became artistic and varied. Materials like ivory, ebony, silver, and gold were added to the iron and early 19th century steel in the manufacture of smaller, more delicate instruments. The compendium of tools grew to include refinements of cutting tools, improved forceps and retractors, fine suture needles, new diagnostic tools, catheters, and probes for visualizing body cavities.[16(pp43–64)] Catheters, endoscopes, and wound drainage devices were made of metal until the 1850s, when Goodyear developed vulcanization of rubber by mixing the raw material from rubber trees with white lead and sulfur. This allowed for the production of rubber sheets and tubing, dramatically changing how important tools surgical tools could be developed for both function and comfort.[2(p126)]

ANTISEPSIS AND ASEPSIS

Surgery became painless in the 1840s, but the threat of life-ending infection remained a critical problem that hindered progress and good outcomes from conservative surgical strategies. In 1847, Semmelweis (1818 to 1865) initiated the concept of prophylactic antisepsis that aimed to prevent the entry of the germs into the wound. He had noted that women attended by midwives, who did not spend time in the dissecting rooms prior to attending women in labor, did not have puerperal fever as often as those cared for by physicians. He demonstrated a dramatic drop in sickness and death on units where physicians thoroughly cleaned their hands, but his findings were not accepted by the surgeons of his day. Later in the century, his concept of keeping germs out of the wound would pave the path for aseptic surgery. In an era where surgery was still limited by the lack of knowledge about how to prevent infection, the work of Semmelweis would eventually open the field for surgery more delicate, complicated, and risky surgery than ever before. This paradigm shift would spur the entire field of surgical instrumentation.[8(pp132–5)]

WAR SURGERY WITHOUT GERM THEORY

It is important to note that in the period between the work of Semmelweiss and that of Pasteur and Lister, two major wars were fought. The Crimean War began in 1854 and lasted 3 years, and the American Civil War was fought from 1861 to 1865. Anesthesia was not always available during these wars, and the human cost in sepsis and communicable diseases was higher than war wounds or battle injuries. Florence Nightingale demonstrated the value of cleanliness and good nutrition in healing injured soldiers and reducing communicable diseases. She worked for reform in the British Army Hospitals in the Crimean War and helped to lower death rates from infection. While the germ theory had not been demonstrated at the time of the war, her insistence on cleanliness and acceptable food made a difference for the soldiers in the overcrowded hospital. Her book, *Notes on Nursing*, was available to many Civil War era nurses. The presence of volunteer and Army nurses in the Civil War provided housekeeping and cleaning assistance that made a difference to the soldiers in many primitive care centers.[8(pp54–80),14(pp121–6)]

The surgical armamentarium for both of these wars included amputation tools such as tourniquets, saws, and ligatures. Surgeons also carried bloodletting instruments, scissors, needles, and knives. Many of the surviving recollections of Civil War nurses and the historical analysis of this era give no mention of nurses caring for the surgical equipment or instruments. In these pregerm theory conflicts, surgeons cared for their tools, because they were considered valuable and hard to replace. This was the post-anesthesia era marked by creative, artistic surgical tools made of valuable materials.

The many tool sets ordered by the military came from skilled manufacturers and often were housed in expensive hardwood cases lined with velvet. The primary surgery in both of these conflicts was amputation, often without anesthesia, and the status of surgeons dropped significantly because of the sudden need for staff and limited numbers of skilled, properly trained practitioners. Histories reveal the use of surgeons without any medical training being forced to fill the role after major battles.[5(pp177–86),8(pp54–80),16(p58),19(pp1–6),20(p125)]

Pasteur (1822 to 1895), a chemist, worked for years to demonstrate the presence of germs and their role in disease in people. His research began with animals and built upon earlier work of Semmelweis and Jenner (smallpox vaccination). Physicians who still believed in the spontaneous generation of diseases initially challenged his ideas. He finally demonstrated the destruction of microorganisms in milk, and the process of pasteurization bears his name. He also demonstrated the value of immunization against infectious diseases. In 1885, he successfully immunized a child who had been bitten by a rabid animal, and the child survived. His research preceded the work of Lister (1827 to 1912), who recognized the value of his theory.[3(pp554–7),8(pp128–34)]

Lister's antiseptic approach aimed to eliminate germs in the operating room by spraying a mist of carbolic acid and by irrigating wounds with antiseptic solutions of carbolic acid. Lister described his observations and noted that closed fractures healed without infection, while compound fractures that broke skin developed pus. He believed that infection was caused by disease-causing dust that was in the air. The process of antisepsis included the scrubbing of hands with strong soap, and soaking in solutions of carbolic acid was also used in this attempt to remove germs from the operating suite. Lister came to Philadelphia in 1876 and convinced a few surgeons to try his approach; the outcomes were excellent. This stimulated the period of antisepsis that aimed to clean the surgical suite to prevent entry of infections and then to wash away infection with chemicals toxic to whatever was causing the pus. Although the work of Pasteur and Lister was aimed at preventing or managing infection from microorganisms, a by-product of their discoveries was an entire new age of surgical instrumentation manufacture and maintenance. The age of artistic surgical instruments with their carved handles and elegant scissors came to an abrupt end.[16(p71)]

MODERN GERM-FREE TOOLS

A new generation of tools and equipment was developed to provide antisepsis in surgery. The growth of antisepsis with its corrosive compounds and then aseptic technique that demanded boiling instruments doomed the artistic tools that had been so popular after the discovery of anesthesia. Surgeons needed less-ornate tools that could be taken apart for more thorough cleaning. Scissors, knife handles, forceps, and other multiple-part instruments had to be made of steel and noncorrosive metals.[2(pp13–4),16(p141)]

A sampling of catalogs for surgical instruments from the late 19th century reveals how quickly the field of manufacturing and specialization occurred as surgery became both painless and less risky for postoperative infections. For example, the George Teimann Company advertised over 700 pages of surgical equipment and supplies for 12 specialties and major or minor procedures. Every type of clamp, needle, forceps, retractor, and irrigator was listed for orthopedics, ophthalmology, or obstetric cases. This was one of many catalogs available and was a dramatic improvement over the few pages of surgical wares formerly offered by drug and medical supply houses in the early part of the century.[16(pp64–72),21]

The development of the one piece of equipment that touches nursing most intimately might be dubbed the love story and the rubber gloves. In 1889, Halstead, surgeon at The Johns Hopkins Hospital, requested the Goodyear Rubber Company to create two pairs of rubber gloves with gauntlets for his operating room scrub nurse, Ms Hampton, a member of the first graduating class in the new training school at the hospital. She had developed an allergic rash from the harsh corrosive sublimate hand rinse. She was the first person known to use sterilized rubber gloves. A year later she became Mrs Halstead. This story, while touching, also demonstrates that nurses had made their way into the operating room as assistants and managers of care. Students in the early training schools in this country cared for hospital equipment, including surgical instruments, and more than half of the curriculum and practice time addressed patient needs in various types of surgeries. Unlike the Civil War volunteers, the nurses in the closing years of century were contributing members of the surgical team and no longer relegated to household duties as they had been in the 1860s. Soon after this first demonstration, surgeons began wearing the gloves, bringing surgery closer to the asepsis that was needed.[17(p475)]

The 1890s have been characterized as a period of radical surgery when new innovative surgeries were developed in many specialties with the aid of the acceptance of aseptic heat-based techniques and painless procedures. Sterile fields and mass production of even the most delicate instruments brought innovative surgery into many regions of the country. Specialization continued to grow in popularity, and surgeons began to focus on specific types of surgery in great numbers. Although the problem of hemorrhage and blood replacement still remained, it was possible to perform procedures not feasible prior to this era. Elective surgery grew, and many procedures were attempted, such as the appendectomy, prior to the patient being in dire straits.[16(p13)]

20TH CENTURY INNOVATIONS AND WARS

The 20th century was a period of refinement of surgical instrumentation. Two innovations changed the basic tools of surgery the most. First, the development of stainless steel in 1913 enabled manufacturers to develop truly corrosion- and rust-proof instruments that would endure for longer periods. Also, the development of plastics, starting with Bakelite in 1907, led to the changes that surgeons have come to expect in tools formerly fashioned out of or cushioned with rubber. The growth of disposable equipment also has dramatically changed surgery in the past century.[2(pp119,127)]

These innovations spurred an explosion in instrumentation experimentation and refinement. Before the World War I, many instruments that had been fashioned in the 1890s were refined and developed for mass use. Some of these tools were used in the war (1914 to 1918). Others were in the design phase but used and refined as the result of learning from war experiences just as the surgeons had done in the Middle Ages.[9(pp138–47),10(pp14–22),22(pp55–69)]

Unfortunately, the past century saw many major and minor wars that have been credited with surgical technique and instrumentation advances. Expediency is often the stimulus for rapid change, and World War I created great human need for surgical innovation. Wounds were caused by high-explosive, high-velocity missiles, machine gun bullets, shell fragments, and shrapnel, and created more physical damage than ever before. The wounds were dirty, and this was the era before antibiotics. Many patients died of gangrene in spite of aggressive amputation. New orthopedic devices and prostheses were developed to meet the needs of these trauma victims. New splints such as the Thomas splint were introduced to prevent compound fractures during treatment. Cushing (1869 to 1939) developed new neurosurgical procedures for treating head trauma. He used electromagnets to remove metal bodies from brains. Many experiments were done to cope with blood loss, but hemorrhage still claimed many victims. Toward the end of the war, sodium citrate was discovered to be a stable anticoagulant, making blood storage possible. The high number of facial injuries in the war stimulated plastic surgery innovations and research.[2(p12),9(pp138–45)]

This was the first war where trained, registered nurses were active in the military and American Red Cross Hospitals throughout the war theater. Nurses described their experiences with the surgical patients in great detail in nursing journals. The key roles and functions that they played related to support and assistance in the operating rooms, sterilization of instruments, and care of the numerous bandages that were part of postoperative care. Nursing often made the difference for surgical patients in this last war to be fought without antibiotics. Meticulous asepsis in the operating room and in postoperative care was critical for survival. Proper care of the surgical instruments under the austere and crude war conditions of this era was a nursing role that provided for patient survival. These nurses suffered many deprivations as the result of their war nursing but emphasized the value of the cleanliness and pain relief that they were able to bring the patients.[8(pp349–60)]

World War II enabled surgeons to consolidate many of the trauma techniques begun in World War I. The demands of war promoted the use of penicillin, and surgeons developed innovative burn surgeries. Blood transfusion techniques were improved, and dried plasma was developed. Surgeons were able to treat patients more rapidly as evacuation procedures were improved, and field hospitals were moved closer to the point of injury. Instruments that had been developed and refined in World War I were available to teams in the military and voluntary hospitals. Entire hospital units were formed from many of the larger hospitals in the United States and took their surgeons, equipment, and technology to the war theaters around the world. Nurses were better trained, and all branches of the military had developed experienced nursing units. Surgical nurses moved with their units and provided support in the operating room while caring for postoperative patients who were recovering from much more sophisticated surgeries aimed at preserving function as well as lives. This was also the first war where air transport became a means for evacuating injured soldiers out of the conflict area. Nurses went with those soldiers, providing postsurgical care during long journeys and often had to provide emergency support en route.[2(p12),8(pp510–41),9(p147)]

The second half of the 20th century was a period of refinement of earlier discoveries and pathfinding surgeries that pushed the limits of known interventions. Open heart surgeries became possible because of heart bypass technology. The entire field of transplantation and tissue replacement grew because of advances in understanding of human immune response and tissue management. The instrumentation continued to advance with the development of lighter, stronger metals such as titanium. The creation of fiberoptics has changed endoscopic tools, and as the surgery has become more cell-specific, the miniaturization of tools and use of magnification tools have grown. Orthopedic tools that permit many types of arthroscopic surgery have helped surgeons to return function to joints. Thoracoscopy, although first introduced in 1910, has advanced to include video-assisted procedures using stapling technology. Laparoscopic surgery prompted the development of new tubular instruments, allowing for greater access to internal organs with minimal incisions.[2(pp35,141),10(pp39–40)]

Other issues have been addressed in the 20th century, such as the technical issue of operating on lungs using an open incision. The problem of pneumothorax when attempting to operate on a lung was a technical issue studied and worked on for years. Once the problem of ventilation and aeration during surgery was solved, the variety of procedures and growth of instruments grew dramatically. Many varieties of thoracic tools used today began as innovations either before or after this technical problem was solved.[10(pp14–44)]

A LOOK TO THE FUTURE

The issue of disposable tools that are costly is one that will have to be addressed in the future. With the continued development of plastics and other synthetic materials, many modern labor-saving tools, such as automatic wound closure instruments that are thrown away after one use, may or may not survive long-term when costs and environmental issues are considered. Disposability grew in popularity in the 1960s but may be reconsidered in some cases with the increasing environmental and cost sensibilities of this century. Other changes on the horizon are hard to grasp but probably no more outlandish than the idea that germs one cannot see with the eye could make one sick. How would a surgeon of 1910 have responded to the idea that catheters made of modern materials could be threaded through an artery and atherosclerotic plaque be compressed to relieve heart pain? The use of robotics in the operating suite for specific procedures is a reality and growing in application. The current trend toward minimally invasive surgery will continue to grow, with fewer and fewer sites open to incision. Surgical interventions on fetuses in the womb, microsurgeries on tiny blood vessels, and a myriad of neurosurgical and ophthalmologic procedures may stimulate the invention of new instrumentation. One expert has proposed the idea that lasers and use of sound or other waves may one day make surgical instruments obsolete. This time is still in the future.[16(p8),23–25]

SO WHAT?

No history or overview is complete without asking this question: How does this study of history relate to the fast-paced practice that surgeons and nurses have today? First, as Kirkup noted in his germinal work on the history of surgical instruments, advances in surgical tools have to be ongoing if the transitions to new paradigms will be possible. Although there was seemingly slow progress in surgical instrumentation before the discovery of anesthesia, there had been a beginning in specialty instruments and experimentation with different types of materials used in tool manufacture that set the stage for the explosion of instrument production that followed that discovery.[2(pix)]

Each discovery tends to lead to a shift in needs for tools or instruments to implement them, such as the specialized clamps that vascular surgery demands. Research stimulates change. Nurses today are much more heavily committed to research and to solving clinical problems, and they need to understand this process of discovery and change. Second, progress will someday make what is done today seem as antiquated as using a fingernail as a knife or scalpel. There is always room to improve, innovate, and recreate better strategies for patients and their changing needs, but one must remember the past. The recognition of previous innovation is critical to the future. As one surgeon reminded his peers, "The young surgeon nourished on surgical history will be more rounded intellectually, more stimulated as a thinker, and generally better prepared to care for the surgical patient."[26(p2)] The same could be said of nurses. Finally, looking back enables one to find heroes. Heroes are people who have persevered or were the pathfinders for those seeking to improve what is done for the safety and well being of this generation. Everyone needs heroes; perhaps the reader has found one or two in this fascinating saga.

ACKNOWLEDGMENTS

The author wishes to thank Dr David Juergens, librarian, director of collection development at Rowland Medical Library of the University of Mississippi Medical Center, for his assistance and collaboration in the data collection for this article. Also author acknowledges the assistance of N. Kenneth Nail Jr, Assistant Professor of Archives and History at University of Mississippi Medical Center in Jackson during the preparation of the manuscript.

REFERENCES

1. Nutting MA, Dock L. History of nursing: the evolution of nursing systems from earliest times to the foundation of the first English and American training schools for nurses, vol. 1. New York: GP Putnam and Sons; 1935.
2. Kirkup J. The evolution of surgical instruments: an illustrated history from ancient times to the twentieth century. Novato (CA): Norman Science Surgery Series; 2006.
3. Lyons A, Petrucelli RJ. Medicine: an illustrated history. New York: Harry Abrams; 1978.
4. Rifkinson-Mann S. Cranial surgery in ancient Peru. In: Anderson R, editor. Sources in the history of medicine. Upper Saddle River (NJ): Pearson Prentice Hall; 2007. p. 7–10.
5. Dolan J. Nursing in society. Philadelphia: W.B. Saunders; 1973.
6. The Edwin Smith papyrus. In: Anderson R, editor. Sources in the history of medicine. Upper Saddle River (NJ): Pearson Prentice Hall; 2007. p. 25–6.
7. Haeger K. The illustrated history of surgery. New York: Bell Publishing Company; 1988.
8. Kalisch P, Kalisch B. The advance of American nursing. 2nd edition. Boston: Little Brown and Company; 1986.
9. Ellis H. A history of surgery. Cambridge (MA): Cambridge University Press; 2001.
10. Hagopian E, Mann C, Galibet L, et al. The history of thoracic surgical instruments and instrumentation. Chest Surg Clin N Am 2000;10(1):9–43.
11. Felter R, West D. Surgical nursing. Philadelphia: F.A. Davis; 1940.
12. Hibbard B. The obstetrician's armamentarium: historical obstetric instruments and their inventors. San Anselmo (CA): Norman Publishing; 2000.
13. Dock L, Stewart I. A short history of nursing: from earliest times to the present day. New York: G.P. Putnam's Sons; 1938.
14. Dossey B. Florence nightingale: mystic, visionary, healer. Springhouse (PA): Springhouse; 2000.
15. Brieger GA. Portrait of surgery: surgery in America, 1875-1889. Surg Clin North Am 1987;6(6):1181–216.
16. Edmonson J. American surgical instruments: an illustrated history of their manufacture and a directory of instrument makers to 1900. San Francisco (CA): Norman Publishing; 1997.
17. Wangensteen O, Wangensteen S. The rise of surgery from empiric craft to scientific discipline. Minneapolis (MN): University of Minnesota Press; 1978.
18. Christianson E. Medicine in New England. In: Leavitt J, Numbers R, editors. Sickness and health in America: readings in the history of medicine and public health. Madison (WI): University of Wisconsin Press; 1997.
19. Dammann GA. Pictorial encyclopedia of civil war medical instruments and equipment. Missoula (MT): Pictorial Histories Publishing; 1983.

20. Grace W. The army surgeon's manual. San Francisco (CA): Norman Publishing; 1992.
21. Edmonson J, Hambrecht FT, editors. American armamentarium chiurgicum 1889, centennial edition. San Francisco (CA): Norman Publishing Company; 1989.
22. Bellamy R. History of surgery for penetrating chest trauma. Chest Surg Clin N Am 2000;10(1):55–70.
23. Raman JD, Scott DJ, Cadeddu JA, et al. Role of magnetic anchors during laparo-endoscopic single site surgery and notes. J Endourol 2009;28(5):780–2.
24. Azizkhan R. Lasers in pediatric surgery. Surg Clin North Am 1992;72(6):1315–31.
25. Munker R. Laser blepharoplasty and periorbital laser skin resurfacing. Facial Plast Surg 2001;17(3):209–17.
26. Wilkins E. Why history is important for thoracic surgeons. Chest Surg Clin N Am 2000;10(1):1–7.

Instrument Readiness: A Patient Safety Issue

Patricia Ann Hercules, RN, MS[a,b],*

KEYWORDS

- Instrument readiness • Patient safety • Safe surgery
- Operating room procedures

Susan Albright was a patient in a small community hospital. Daniel Stevens was a patient in a large medical center hospital. Susan was scheduled for a left arthroscopy with meniscus repair. Daniel was scheduled for a right laparoscopic nephrectomy. Their experiences somewhat mirrored each other.

In the small and large hospital, the operating room (OR) team performed the preprocedure verification process, the site was marked, and the time out was performed immediately before starting the procedure. The go sign was given, the procedure began, and the team went into streamlined action.

Susan's surgeon, Dr Azi, was well into the procedure. He was fast and precise. A stab incision was made, the irrigation cannula and trocar inserted, normal saline added, the joint distended, and light source and video camera were connected to the scope. There was no light and it seemed the camera was not working. In fact, the fiberoptic cord had been twisted and tightly coiled and some filaments frayed so that light was not transmitted. There was no other scope available and Susan was awakened, only to be rescheduled for another day.

Daniel's surgeon, Dr Lewis, was also well recognized in the community as swift and compassionate, and he had quality outcomes with his patients. The team enjoyed working with him because he was confident and shared his knowledge. Daniel's laparoscopic nephrectomy included a cystoscopy with placement of a renal balloon catheter, a ureteral catheter, and a Foley urethral catheter. A laparotomy open setup was immediately available just in case the laparoscopy was not successful. This was the case with Daniel. Dr Lewis had already performed the cystoscopy and placed the catheters under fluoroscopy with a C-arm. When Dr Lewis realized that an open procedure was needed, he discontinued the laparoscopic approach and called for the open procedure protocol. This included the appropriate instrument sets and equipment. The instrument pan on the ring stand that was labeled "lap set" was opened, only to find a bone set with chisels, screws, and a drill. There was dead

[a] 2406 Meadow Way, Missouri City, TX 77459, USA
[b] System Clinical Education, Memorial Hermann Healthcare System, Houston, TX, USA
* Corresponding author. 2406 Meadow Way, Missouri City, Texas 77459.
E-mail address: patriciaannhp@gmail.com

Perioperative Nursing Clinics 5 (2010) 15–25
doi:10.1016/j.cpen.2009.11.004
1556-7931/10/$ – see front matter © 2010 Elsevier Inc. All rights reserved.

silence in the room and quite a bit of scurry. There had been a mistake somewhere in the process involving cleaning, disinfecting, assembling, packaging, and, finally, labeling of the set. A sterile lap set was not immediately available and ready. In fact, securing one required a call and a trip to the central sterile processing department. In the interim, Daniel began showing electrocardiogram changes and his blood pressure dropped to a hypotensive level. Even though the anesthesiologist stabilized Daniel, Dr Lewis became anxious with the wait. It was simply taking too much time, as he learned that the OR case volume that day had been heavy and a set had to be sterilized for use. After a considerable length of time, the decision was made to reschedule Daniel when he was more stable. He was awakened and transported to the postoperative care unit for close observation.

The scenarios with Susan and Daniel are hypothetical, but they could have been real. They could be just as real as the following scenarios:

- An elderly male patient was admitted for a right total-knee replacement. A left femoral component (should have been the right one) was handed to the circulating nurse, then to the scrub tech, and then passed to the surgeon. The wrong replacement was not discovered until near the end of the procedure. The surgeon left the right femoral component in the knee because it was tracking well and he believed that removal would cause more damage to the femur.
- The grabber from a laparoscopy set had a crack in the plastic sleeve that covered the end of the instrument. It cracked further and a piece broke off in the patient. The surgeon was unable to locate the entire piece, and had to close the patient, knowing that a foreign body had been retained. After investigation, it was found that the instrument had probably been cracked for quite some time and attention had not been paid to the repair or replacement.
- A female patient with metastatic ovarian cancer was admitted through the emergency room with nausea and vomiting. She was transported to the OR for a vascular access catheter placement. This was done successfully. After the procedure was completed, the circulating nurse noticed that the sterilizer indicator from the tray was not turned and the tray was unsterile.

Lack of instrument readiness was the culprit in each of the above scenarios.

INSTRUMENT READINESS DEFINED

Instrument readiness is a term used to verify that the instruments or associated equipment, or both, are immediately available, functional, sterile if entering the surgical field, and ready for use when the surgical team is ready. For example, if the equipment is a drill set, then included in being ready is verification that the drill set has all the component parts (eg, attachments, power cords, and batteries) and is functional. If it is a set of instruments, then included in being ready is a confirmed count and assurance that scissors can cut, clamps can clamp, retractors can retract, and so forth. If it is an implant, then being ready means providing the correct implant for the patient. If being ready relates to a system, as in laparoscopic or robotic equipment, all component parts must be accounted for, in place, tested, and operationally sound. This verification requires knowledge and accountability on the part of the perioperative nurse and other team members. It also requires an environment in which a culture of safety is a priority. Lack of readiness can lead to questions such as: are patients really safe in the OR?

At the New York State Patient Safety Conference in 2007, John R. Clarke, MD (Professor of Surgery, Drexel University; Clinical Director for Patient Safety, ECRI; and Clinical Director PA Patient Safety Reporting System), asked the same question in a presentation made at the Safety Conference. Dr Clarke's presentation ("Is My Patient Safe in the Operating Room?") identified at-risk behaviors in the OR and OR-adverse events or errors causing delays under anesthesia. The behaviors that were identified included not checking equipment before surgery, multitasking, using electrosurgical equipment in an oxygen-rich environment, unannounced substitutions in the middle of the case, and closing before the final sponge and instrument count. Adverse events causing anesthesia delays were attributed to the surgeon running two rooms; the surgeon being educated on how to use new equipment; needed equipment not available, especially when they were known ahead of time; and other surgeon-related events.[1]

In 2007, the Department of Veterans Affairs, Office of the Inspector General, released a report titled "Review of Patient Safety in the Operating Room in Veterans Health Administration [VHA] Facilities." The report was the result of an inspection of eight VHA medical faculties from October 2005 to May 2006. The purpose of the inspection was to assess and ensure patient safety in the OR. The focus was in three areas:

- Effective policies, procedures, and guidelines to ensure patient safety in the OR.
- The presence of surgical improvement programs to identify problem areas needing improvement.
- Coordination between supply, processing, and distribution (SPD) and the OR[2].

The findings related to SPD coordination with the OR showed that in 25% of the facilities the instrument trays or surgical case carts contained instruments that were broken or incorrect and, in some instances, instruments were missing. One of the facilities had supply shortages and situations in which the OR was receiving contaminated instruments.[2]

Coordination between the SPD and the OR has perhaps one of the greatest impacts on the readiness of instruments and equipment for any surgical procedure. The workflow in the SPD should be one that provides "continuous flow of processed sterile and non-sterile supplies, instruments, and equipment to the ORs."[2] When the process is broken at any point, there is an opportunity for supplies to be unavailable; for instruments to be missing, broken, or incorrect; and for contaminated instruments to be inadvertently used during a procedure. This was the case as stated in the VHA report. Facilities attributed the cause to an unknowledgeable staff and to overall minimal attention to the process.[2]

When the issues were further explored, it was found that the ORs were using creative work-arounds and substitutions to correct the availability issues:

- For the missing, broken, and incorrect instrument issue, it was found that some of the instruments were those most frequently used. These were then fetched from extra supplies.[2]
- In other situations and with specialized instruments, such as the scopes for laparoscopy procedures, it was found that these sometimes came to the OR with mismatched parts. It was acknowledged that if the scopes came from different suppliers, interchanging them would not work.[2]
- When the incidents of contaminated instruments were reviewed, it was found that the OR staff had received instrument trays that were contaminated and that they returned them to the SPD for decontamination and sterilization.

Contamination can occur because debris such as bone fragments remains in the grooves of the instruments, indicating improper cleaning and decontamination procedures.[2]

The summary report from the VHA facilities stated that there were no patient care incidents because the OR staff ensured that the surgical procedures began without the impending issues that were identified. These were corrected before the procedures began. The report of no incidents was good news, and the issues were addressed through process improvement plans.[2] If the staff members had not been so careful, however, patient safety would have been unnecessarily jeopardized.

The report from the VA Office of Inspector General supports lack of instrument readiness as a hurdle that exists in many ORs and again brings to the surface the questions: are our patients at risk in the operating room and should we focus our attention more on instrument readiness as a best practice standard for safe patient care?

HISTORICAL REVIEW OF PATIENT SAFETY
Institute of Medicine Report, November 1999

There has been concentrated attention on patient safety in the operating room for a solid decade now through numerous alarming reports that have spread through the nation and the world. In particular, since the Institute of Medicine (IOM) published "To Err is Human: Building a Safer Health System" in November 1999,[3] issues of patient safety and healthcare errors have captured the attention of the healthcare industry, consumers, the public, and the media. There has been an unearthing of the stories of healthcare errors that have astounded the listener and encouraged the silent to speak out. Subsequently, publicizing the outcomes of errors has provided groundwork for carefully designed plans, regulations, and practice standards that have encouraged learning from mistakes and preventing them in the future. According to the IOM report, mistakes have been many and the causes fell into the categories of diagnostic, treatment, preventive, and other. The latter category includes failure to communicate, equipment failure, and other system failure.[3,4] The inclusion of equipment failure in this category suggests that equipment and, by extension, instrumentation, is critical to the safety and protection of patients undergoing surgical intervention.

Recommendations from the IOM report addressed the causes of errors with recommendations that included establishing a national focus to increase the knowledge base about safety, learning from errors with reporting systems, raising performance standards, and implementing safety systems to ensure safe practices at the point of service.[3]

Sentinel Event Alerts, National Patient Safety Goals, Universal Protocol

The Joint Commission began addressing wrong site surgery over a decade ago. In the Sentinel Event Alerts, in 1998, there was a publication based on a review of 15 cases that had been reported to the Joint Commission. A follow-up report was published in 2001 and was based on 150 reports of surgical errors and their associated risk factors and root causes.[5]

According to the Sentinel Event Alerts, the factors contributing to the increased risk for wrong site, wrong person, or wrong procedure surgery fell into the following categories:

- 19% emergency cases
- 16% physical characteristics that were unusual, including obesity or physical deformities

- 13% time pressure to complete the procedures
- 13% unusual equipment or set-ups in the operating room
- 13% multiple surgeons involved in the cases
- 10% multiple procedures performed during the surgery.[5]

The Sentinel Events Alerts encouraged insight into causes of medical errors and led to the introduction of the time-out procedure that was approved by the Joint Commission in July 2003. It became effective in July 2004 in the 2003–2004 National Patient Safety Goals. In the Joint Commission's Universal Protocol for Preventing Wrong Site, Wrong Procedure, Wrong Person Surgery, the time out was required as an integral step in all operative and other invasive procedures conducted in the OR and other settings that expose patients to more than a minimal risk.[6,7]

The time-out procedure and the Universal Protocol standards as issued by the Joint Commission have made a difference. It has become obvious that the public is aware of the media reports, and consumers' awareness has been raised when they are scheduled for surgery or other invasive procedures. It is also obvious that health care professionals have developed a consciousness and openness to developing and practicing interventions to ensure safe surgery for their patients. As a part of the time-out and Universal Protocol procedures, instrument and equipment availability and functionality are being recognized as important factors in assuring a safe surgical environment.

World Health Organization

The World Health Organization (WHO) "is the directing and coordinating authority for health within the United Nations system. It is responsible for providing leadership on global health matters, shaping the health research agenda, setting norms and standards, articulating evidence-based policy options, providing technical support to countries and monitoring and assessing health trends."[8]

In this capacity, the WHO entered into global initiatives to address the challenge of surgical safety and created the Second Global Patient Safety Challenge: Safe Surgery Saves Lives. A press release by the WHO on June 25, 2008, stated, "With major surgery now occurring at a rate of 234 million procedures per year—one for every 25 people—and studies indicating that a significant percentage result in preventable complications and deaths, WHO today launched a new safety checklist for surgical teams to use in operating theaters, as part of a major drive to make surgery safer around the world."[9]

The World Alliance for Patient Safety, comprising international experts on safety, began work on the Challenge in January 2007 with four areas of focus: infection prevention, safe anesthesia, safe surgical teams, and measurement of surgical services. This group suggested that meeting this challenge could be accomplished in several ways, but, in particular, they identified a very simple set of surgical safety standards in a checklist that would be applicable to all countries and settings for use in operating rooms. They also set in place plans to evaluate this checklist at pilot sites in the WHO regions worldwide.[8]

The Surgical Safety Checklist (**Fig. 1**) identifies key safety steps in surgical intervention that should be implemented in three phases. The steps are: the sign-in phase, before anesthesia is induced; the time-out phase, the period following induction but before the incision; and the sign-out phase, the time during or immediately after wound closure but before the patient leaves the OR.[10]

It is clear that sterile, functional, and available instruments and equipment are essential for safety in the time-out and sign-out phases of the patient's experience in the OR. To anticipate critical events in the time-out phase, the nursing team reviews

SURGICAL SAFETY CHECKLIST (First Edition)

World Health Organization

Before induction of anaesthesia ▶▶▶▶▶▶▶▶   Before skin incision ▶▶▶▶▶▶▶▶▶▶▶▶▶▶   Before patient leaves operating room

SIGN IN

☐ PATIENT HAS CONFIRMED
  • IDENTITY
  • SITE
  • PROCEDURE
  • CONSENT

☐ SITE MARKED/NOT APPLICABLE

☐ ANAESTHESIA SAFETY CHECK COMPLETED

☐ PULSE OXIMETER ON PATIENT AND FUNCTIONING

DOES PATIENT HAVE A:

KNOWN ALLERGY?
☐ NO
☐ YES

DIFFICULT AIRWAY/ASPIRATION RISK?
☐ NO
☐ YES, AND EQUIPMENT/ASSISTANCE AVAILABLE

RISK OF >500ML BLOOD LOSS (7ML/KG IN CHILDREN)?
☐ NO
☐ YES, AND ADEQUATE INTRAVENOUS ACCESS AND FLUIDS PLANNED

TIME OUT

☐ CONFIRM ALL TEAM MEMBERS HAVE INTRODUCED THEMSELVES BY NAME AND ROLE

☐ SURGEON, ANAESTHESIA PROFESSIONAL AND NURSE VERBALLY CONFIRM
  • PATIENT
  • SITE
  • PROCEDURE

ANTICIPATED CRITICAL EVENTS

☐ SURGEON REVIEWS: WHAT ARE THE CRITICAL OR UNEXPECTED STEPS, OPERATIVE DURATION, ANTICIPATED BLOOD LOSS?

☐ ANAESTHESIA TEAM REVIEWS: ARE THERE ANY PATIENT-SPECIFIC CONCERNS?

☐ NURSING TEAM REVIEWS: HAS STERILITY (INCLUDING INDICATOR RESULTS) BEEN CONFIRMED? ARE THERE EQUIPMENT ISSUES OR ANY CONCERNS?

HAS ANTIBIOTIC PROPHYLAXIS BEEN GIVEN WITHIN THE LAST 60 MINUTES?
☐ YES
☐ NOT APPLICABLE

IS ESSENTIAL IMAGING DISPLAYED?
☐ YES
☐ NOT APPLICABLE

SIGN OUT

NURSE VERBALLY CONFIRMS WITH THE TEAM:

☐ THE NAME OF THE PROCEDURE RECORDED

☐ THAT INSTRUMENT, SPONGE AND NEEDLE COUNTS ARE CORRECT (OR NOT APPLICABLE)

☐ HOW THE SPECIMEN IS LABELLED (INCLUDING PATIENT NAME)

☐ WHETHER THERE ARE ANY EQUIPMENT PROBLEMS TO BE ADDRESSED

☐ SURGEON, ANAESTHESIA PROFESSIONAL AND NURSE REVIEW THE KEY CONCERNS FOR RECOVERY AND MANAGEMENT OF THIS PATIENT

THIS CHECKLIST IS NOT INTENDED TO BE COMPREHENSIVE. ADDITIONS AND MODIFICATIONS TO FIT LOCAL PRACTICE ARE ENCOURAGED.

Fig. 1. Surgical safety checklist. (*Courtesy of* the World Health Organization, with permission.)

and assures sterility results and directly inquires about equipment issues or concerns. Knowing that equipment issues, including instruments, are ongoing and rarely unique to any one operating room, it becomes critical that any malfunctioning piece of equipment (eg, electrical drill, endoscope, stapling device, cutting or clamping device) be identified and removed from future use until repaired and made functional. This ongoing review of equipment and instrumentation should be a component of all phases but it culminates in the sign-out phase before instruments and equipment ever leave the operating suite in which the malfunction was discovered.[10]

The Joint Commission Universal Protocol and the WHO Surgical Safety Checklist continue to lead the way for implementation of the recommendations from the IOM report. They are complementary standards, addressing patient safety and focusing on surgical patient safety. The primary focus of the Universal Protocol is to address wrong site, wrong procedure, and wrong person surgery, while the primary focus of the WHO Surgical Safety checklist is to promote all aspects of safe surgery. Of significance to all aspects are readiness and the need for equipment and instrumentation to be functional and immediately available before surgery.[11]

INFLUENCING FACTORS: READINESS AND SAFETY
Availability

The patient signs the operative permit for surgery, agreeing to have a body part opened and excised or repaired. In doing so, the patient places himself or herself in the hands of the surgical team and with confidence that the surgical outcome does not hinge on instrument availability. In fact, it would probably never occur to the patient that sometimes instruments and equipment may not be at the right place at the right time for any patient's particular procedure. It does happen, however, that instrument availability is an issue in most ORs and, in fact, it is frequently high on the list of process improvement programs in perioperative surgical suites. Process improvement becomes a real key because the availability of surgical instruments does not depend on the individual actions of one person. The scramble for instruments immediately before a procedure remains a common scenario.[12]

Instrument availability was high on the list of issues from the Department of Veteran Affairs in the report titled "Review of Patient Safety in the Operating room in Veterans Health Administrations Facilities."[2] It also caused an issue at the Toledo Hospital, Toledo, Ohio. Toledo Hospital performs an average of 70 to 80 procedures a day and possesses over 1400 instrument sets and thousands of single-item instruments. A process improvement study was initiated to identify and correct the issues, as the preliminary data revealed that "instruments were available only 64% of the time, so in 36% of the procedures, problems with instrument availability were experienced."[12] These problems were due to trends such as errors in the instrument tray set-ups, missing instruments from sets, issues with tracking instrument loss, poor communication between departments, no regular repair schedules, and poorly trained staff. The staff of this hospital tackled each issue to bring about resolution and put into place a system to move past this hurdle.[12]

Substitutions

When instruments are not available, there is a tendency for substitutions or make-do practices. The patient may not sustain injury or harm but, conversely, the patient may not be so lucky and become at risk for surgical error. The following is an example of lack of availability leading to substitutions that resulted in surgical error.

Perioperative grand rounds provide a time to discuss incidents and solutions for patients undergoing surgical intervention. One such incident was discussed in the Perioperative Grand Rounds Section of the *AORN Journal*, based on original publication in the Agency for Healthcare Research and Quality's "Case and Commentary:"[13,14]

> *The patient was scheduled for an elective hysteroscopy and dilatation and curettage. When the patient was in the OR and prepared for the surgery, it was noticed that the hysteroscopy set was unavailable—not yet sterilized because of earlier use in the day. Therefore a "makeshift" hysteroscopy set was created and used. The patient had a cardiac arrest during insufflation of the uterus, was resuscitated, and a day later was discharged. There was analysis of the situation to determine the cause of the cardiac arrest and multiple problems and causative factors were brought forward for discussion. Because, however, the arrest occurred "during insufflation of the uterus," there were questions about whether it could have been caused by air embolism or CO_2 gas embolization. The question also arose about whether or not it could have been caused by the makeshift hysteroscopy equipment that resulted in use of the wrong insufflator, causing the patient to receive an abnormally high flow rate. Another question was posed regarding whether or not the embolus could have been in the hysteroscopic tubing if it had not been purged before use with the patient.*

Again, when instruments are not available, the patient is at risk and the door opens for errors. When this occurs, another door can open—that of stress. Stress has a predominant role in surgical error for it can be not only a stimulus for unsafe practice, but a result of unsafe practice. In other words, when instruments and equipment are not immediately available and ready for use when the surgeon is ready, additional stress among surgical team members is likely to occur and the potential for additional surgical error is likely to occur.

Stress and Unsafe Performance

The perioperative nurses at one institution in northeast Florida were surveyed because of the large amount of stress that seemed to prevail in their environment. A quality improvement team began to look at the extent to which nurses perceived their work to be stressful and to determine the stressors that supported that perception. The top three stressors were patients dying in the OR (48%), pressure to work faster (41%), and equipment that did not work (41%).[15]

Comments made by the nurses led to conclusion that the effect of stress on nurses places them in a balancing act between the organization, the profession, and themselves as persons. The cost of stress is a significant one in terms of health and behavior—to the individual and to the team. Additionally, the situations that produce the stress also have the potential to place the patient at risk for injury. In times of stress, it is easy to overlook a routine or process and move into the realm of potential adverse events or near misses.[15]

Intimidating and disruptive behavior is defined by the Joint Commission as "verbal outbursts and physical threats as well as passive activities such as refusing to perform assigned tasks or quietly exhibiting uncooperative attitudes during routine activities."[16] Root causes of disruptive behaviors were found to stem from individual and process-related factors and are pronounced during times of fatigue and stress.[16] In the operating room, reasons such as productivity, mandates to shorten turnaround time, the drive toward cost containment, daily changes in shifts and the team, lack of interdepartmental support, and unrealistic expectations cause errors in case preparation, readiness, and implementation. This means errors in preparing the necessary supplies and equipment for the case, assuring sterility and functional order, and then making them available at the moment they are needed in surgery. It also influences safe care and handling after surgery so that instruments and equipment are ready and available for subsequent patients.[17]

Distractions, Interruptions, and Fatigue

Readiness is impacted by distractions, interruptions, and fatigue. Perioperative nurses generally agree that these factors are pervasive in the perioperative environment.

A group of researchers observed distractions and interruptions in a large teaching hospital in United Kingdom with 50 general surgery procedures. The disruptions included telephones, pagers, staff member communications, communication difficulties, and equipment-related issues. Through observation, the researchers concluded that the conversations were responsible for the largest number of interruptions, along with pagers, movement, and non–procedure-related conversations. They reported that many of the distractions were related to the equipment, environment, and events relating to the procedure. They also concluded that a large amount of disruption could have a negative impact on OR teamwork and surgical outcomes for the patients.[18]

OR Efficiency, Effectiveness, and Throughput

Streamlined, efficient movement of the patient through the surgical experience contributes to the patient's ongoing comfort and safety. Therefore, processing the flow of care efficiently becomes a benefit for the patient and for the operational efficiency of the OR.

It is well documented that the drive for operational efficiency and effectiveness is a priority in today's economic environment—that is, as long as the quality of care is maintained. Efficiency programs have been targeted as strategies to overcome the issues of on-time starts and turnaround time for efficiency improvement and for the smooth implementation of safe patient care in the surgical environment.

One example of an efficiency program was at Stony Brook Medical Center, Stony Brook, New York. The program addressed on-time starts, patient transfers, turnover time, accuracy of surgeon preference cards, staff performance, and communication about patient needs. The data they gathered about surgeon preference cards revealed that they were handwritten, sporadically updated for the specialty services, and lacked a process to routinely review or measure them for accuracy. Preference cards are specifically intended to meet the surgeon's needs when preparing for the patient's surgery. This includes identifying the right instruments and equipment, and laying the groundwork for them to be immediately available and prepared when the surgeon is ready. Procedure cards that are incorrect and outdated do not guide the nurse who is new to the surgeon or procedure to prepare adequately so that the patient can be safely cared for with the appropriate support for the surgeon. Stony Brook Medical Center achieved success in this aspect of their efficiency program. A process was put in place to assure immediate and ongoing changes to the procedure cards are made so that the required instruments and equipment are prepared when the surgeon is ready.[19]

OR throughput is a name for the process of patient flow through the perioperative experience. The challenge of OR and perioperative leadership is to deliver quality patient care in an efficient and qualitative manner.

A medical center in Southwestern Vermont is not significantly different from other hospitals seeking to improve their patient flow from entry to exit. A Six Sigma team was requested to assist them with gathering data and analyzing all aspects of the point-of-care site for the patient and to assist them with changing their processes for better safe patient care. The OR throughput project began with looking at the scheduling of surgical procedures because they were not meeting surgeon and patient needs. Initially, a survey was distributed to surgical and nursing staff to gather their responses and to identify major themes to the prolonged throughput. It was found that the largest culprit to prolonged throughput was categorized as procedural delay. Other reasons found included excess paperwork, intravenous starts, unstocked rooms, and missing instruments or equipment.[20]

The goal of Southwestern Vermont Medical Center was to improve the quality of the care for the patient through a more effective throughput. In doing so, the intended by-product was to instill in the staff a sense of accomplishment and productivity. When the project was completed, it was observed that the staff demonstrated a greater sense of cohesiveness, pride, and accountability in pursing their initial goal of an enhanced patient throughput.[20]

SUMMARY

In reviewing available data and real-life stories regarding instrument readiness, it is evident that instrument and equipment readiness and availability is needed nationally and internationally to safeguard patient care in the OR. It is also evident that safeguarding the patient leads toward greater efficiency and effectiveness. Therefore, it seems reasonable that the health care profession should take a closer look at equipment and instrument readiness as a patient safety issue.

REFERENCES

1. Clarke JR. Is my patient safe in the operating room? Paper presented at New York state patient Safety Conference. Albany (NY), 2007. Available at: http://www.health.state.ny.us/professionals/patients/patient_safety/conference/2007/. Accessed June 9, 2009.
2. Office of Inspector General. Department of veterans affairs. Review of patient safety in the operating room in veterans health administration facilities. 2007. Available at: http://www.va.gov/oig/54/reports/VAOIG-05-00379-91.pdf. Report No. 05-00379-91. Published. Accessed June 9, 2009.
3. Committee on Quality of Health Care in America. Institute of medicine. To err is human: building a safer health system. Available at: http://www.iom.edu/~/media/Files/Report%20Files/1999/To-Err-is-Human/To%20Err%20is%20Human%201999%20%20report%20brief.ashx. Published November, 1999. Accessed November 30, 2009.
4. Leape L, Lawthers AG, Brennan TA, et al. Preventing medical injury. Qual Rev Bull 1993;19(5):144–9.
5. The Joint Commission. A follow-up review of wrong site surgery. Available at: Sentinel Event Alert 2001;10 http://www.jointcommission.org/SentinelEvents/SentinelEventAlert/sea_24.htm. Published December 5, 2001. Accessed June 9, 2009.
6. The Joint Commission. Universal protocol. Available at: http://www.jointcommission.org/PatientSafety/UniversalProtocol. Updated June 9, 2009. Accessed June 9, 2009.
7. Aorn. ACS, The Joint Commission partner with AORN on National Time Out Day. Available at: http://www.aorn.org/News/May2008News/NTOD2008/. Accessed November 30, 2009.
8. World Health Organization. About WHO. Available at: http://www.who.int/about/en/. Accessed June 9, 2009.

9. World Health Organization. New checklist to help make surgery safer. Available at: http://www.who.int/mediacentre/news/releases/2008/pr20/en/index.html. Published June 25, 2008. Accessed June 9, 2009.

10. World Alliance for Patient Safety. Implementation manual, WHO surgical safety checklist (first edition): safe surgery saves lives. Available at: http://www.who.int/patientsafety/safesurgery/tools_resources/SSSL_Manual_finalJun08.pdf. Accessed June 9, 2009.

11. The Joint Commission. Clarification of universal protocol compliance. This month for physicians 2009;2. Available at: http://www.jointcommission.org/NR/rdonlyres/5425360E-DE36-447C-9779-3307A27A2DEA/0/02_09_this_month_phys.pdf. Accessed June 9, 2009.

12. Prephan L. Surgical instrument availability. AORN J 2005;81(5):1017–22.

13. Girard NJ. Perioperative grand rounds: are the instruments ready? AORN J 2009; 89(1):244, 119.

14. Agency for Healthcare Research and Quality. Case & commentary: making do. Commentary by Bradley, LD. Morbidity and mortality rounds on the web. 2003 Available at: http://www.webmm.ahrq.gov/case.aspx?caseID=28. Accessed June 9, 2009.

15. Kingdon B, Halvorsen F. Perioperative nurses' perceptions of stress in the workplace. AORN J 2006;84(4):507–14.

16. The Joint Commission. Behaviors that undermine a culture of safety. Sentinel Event Alert 2008;40. Available at: http://www.jointcommission.org/SentinelEvents/SentinelEventAlert/sea_40.htm. Accessed June 9, 2009.

17. Beyea SC. Promoting a culture of safety by addressing bad behavior. AORN J 2008;88(4):637–9.

18. Healey AN, Sevdalis N, Vincent CA. Measuring intra-operative interference from distraction and interruption observed in the operating theatre. Ergonomics 2006; 49(5–6):589–604.

19. Scheriff K, Gunderson D, Intelisano A. Implementation of an or efficiency program. AORN J 2008;88(5):775–89.

20. Fairbanks CB. Using six sigma and lean methodologies to improve or throughput. AORN J 2007;86(1):73–82.

Review of Best Practices and Literature on Instrument Counts

Cynthia K. Halvorson, RN, MSN, CNOR

KEYWORDS

- Surgical instrument counts • Sponge/swab • Sharp/needle
- Evidence-based practice • Best practices
- Retained foreign objects • Never-events

With a heightened emphasis on patient safety and a lowered tolerance for the occurrence of "never-events" there is a need for improved practices. Evidence-based knowledge bridges this gap by providing direction for best practices that ensure consistent and sustained safe patient care and optimal outcomes. Perioperative nursing has a long-standing and well-respected position of advocating for safe patient care. With intimate knowledge of the counting process, perioperative nurses, as key stakeholders in the multidisciplinary approach, must contribute to the body of evidence regarding best practices for effective surgical counts.

THE NEED FOR EVIDENCE-SUPPORTED BEST PRACTICES
New Paradigm, New Philosophy

For more than a decade there has been an increasing awareness of medical errors and their potential for causing devastating harm to patients. Multiple patient safety initiatives have been implemented with the intent to identify, prevent, and reduce their occurrence. In response, professional associations, patient safety organizations, regulatory agencies, and governmental departments have developed practice guidelines, position statements, accreditation expectations, and directives (**Tables 1** and **2**).

Several surgical errors, including retained surgical items, are included on the National Quality Forum's Severe Reportable Events list, more commonly known as "never-events."[12] The National Quality Forum defines never-events as preventable adverse events that should never occur; are identifiable and measurable; and are of concern to the public, health care professionals, and providers. Further, never-events are significantly influenced by the policies and procedures of the health care facility. The Centers for Medicare and Medicaid Services include never-events in their

Im Spycher 2, CH 8124 Maur, Switzerland
E-mail address: cynthia_halvorson@yahoo.com

Perioperative Nursing Clinics 5 (2010) 27–44
doi:10.1016/j.cpen.2009.11.003
1556-7931/10/$ – see front matter © 2010 Elsevier Inc. All rights reserved.

Table 1 Professional organizations' recommended practices for surgical counts	
Professional Organization	**Recommended Practice**
Association of Perioperative Registered Nurses (AORN) USA www.aorn.org	Recommended practices for sponge, sharp, and instruments[1]
Australian College of Operating Room Nurses (ACORN) www.acorn.org	S3 counting of accountable items used during surgery[2] Educational guide to familiarize and apply S3[3]
Association for Perioperative Practice (AfPP) UK www.afpp.rog.uk	Managing the risk in swab, instrument, and needle counts[4]
Operating Room Nurses Association of Canada (ORNAC) www.ornac.ca	Surgical counts[5]
South African Theater Nurse (SATS) http://home.mweb.co.za/s./s.a.t.s	Swab, instrument, and needle counts[6]
International Federation of Perioperative Nurses (IFPN) www.ifpn.org.uk	IFPN guideline 1002 for surgical counts: sponges, sharps and instruments[7]
American College of Surgeons (ACS) www.facs.org	ST-51 Statement on the prevention of retained foreign bodies after surgery[8]

classification of hospital-acquired conditions. Hospital-acquired conditions are considered not present on admission and, as such, are no longer reimbursed as a secondary diagnosis by Centers for Medicare and Medicaid Services effective October 1, 2008.[13] Reimbursement has shifted from fee-for-service to pay-for-performance. The Joint Commission includes retained foreign bodies in their reportable sentinel events statistics.[14] This intense focus indicates a heightened emphasis on patient safety and a reduced tolerance for the occurrence of errors.

There is a need to improve health care practices. Clinical practice is evolving from opinion and anecdotal experience-based protocols to evidence-based guidelines. Evidence-based knowledge provides the direction for effective protocols and practices for sustained optimal outcomes.

Surgical Instrument Counts

The initial rationale for conducting instrument counts was based in inventory control.[15] It was not until 1976 that the Association of Perioperative Registered Nurses first published the "Standards for Sponge, Needle, and Instrument Procedures."[16] The introduction of that document discusses patient safety as the intent of the standard. The current "Recommended Practices for Sponge, Sharp, and Instrument Counts" stresses that the intended primary outcome is to ensure that the patient is free from harm caused by extraneous objects (ie, retained surgical items, including instruments).[1]

When a surgical count fails to prevent a retained surgical instrument, four areas of risk are presented: (1) safety, (2) reputation, (3) legal, and (4) financial. Patient safety is severely compromised, with significant morbidity and mortality resulting. Professional reputation of the facility and involved practitioners can suffer. The legal domain neither mandates that counts be performed, nor prescribes specifics of the process itself.[1] The expectation is that no instruments are left behind. The mere presence of a retained instrument speaks for itself (the doctrine of res ipsa loquitur), making the occurrence virtually nondefensible.[17] These three risks have a threefold financial impact: (1) the cost of the event (loss of reimbursement); (2) indemnity payment to the patient; and (3) legal defense fees. The challenge is to develop and consistently implement, monitor, and evaluate best practices to ensure intended outcomes.

Table 2
Guidelines, directives, and protocols for surgical counts

Organization	Document	Comment
World Health Organization (WHO) www.who.int	Objective 7: the team will prevent inadvertent retention of instruments or sponges in surgical wounds[9]	Consistent with the recommendations of international perioperative nursing associations
Veterans Health Administration (VHA) www.va.gov	VHA Directive 2006–030 Prevention of Retained Surgical Items[10]	Includes detailed methodic wound exploration steps Components of instrument system counted individually Suggested additional strategies Standardized orientation to counting Protocol for new physicians and nurses Minimize personnel changes
Institute for Clinical System Improvement (ICSI) www.icsi.org	Health Care Protocol: Prevention of Unintentionally Retained Foreign Objects in Surgery[11]	Evidence-based guideline with annotated algorithm of count procedures from room set-up to end of case, including count discrepancy protocol Includes definitions, detailed radiograph imaging protocol for count discrepancies; parallel process and "Red Rules"

FINDING THE EVIDENCE FOR SURGICAL INSTRUMENT COUNT BEST PRACTICE
Literature Search

This literature review identifies current research studies (medical and nursing) on surgical instrument counts; reviews research evidence supporting best practices for surgical instrument counts; and discusses implications and recommendations of study findings. Multiple keywords were used in the literature search, including "surgical counts," "surgical instrument counts," "sponge-swab," "sharp-needle," "instrument counts," "retained foreign object-body-item," and "retained surgical instrument." The literature search was conducted during May and June 2009 using the PubMed and CINAHL databases for citations published between 2003 and 2009. The reference lists of selected studies provided additional citations. Also searched were Web sites for professional associations (nursing and medical), patient safety organizations, regulatory agencies, and governmental departments (federal) for position statements, recommended practices, and accreditation expectations.

Criteria used to select citations in this literature review included articles reporting primary research related to surgical counts in general and surgical instruments in particular. Literature reviews of studies on surgical counts were also included. International studies were included. Articles discussing sponge-swab and sharp-needle counting protocols only, editorial comments, and single or unusual occurrence case reports were excluded. The limits to this literature review include one reviewer (the author) of a limited number of studies, which are not exclusive or specific to instrument counts.

Search Results

Limited literature

Despite the significant volume of discussion on surgical never-events, few studies exploring best practices for surgical count protocols have been published. The identified studies investigated all three categories of countable items (sponge, sharp, instrument). No studies were found that addressed surgical instruments exclusively; however, one discussion of instrument counts was extracted from a review of studies.[18] Fourteen primary research studies were identified from the literature search, of which 11 were from the medical domain and 3 from the nursing domain. International studies included three medical (Turkey, Russia) and the three nursing (Germany, Australia) studies.

Final selection

Final studies included five medical (United States) and three nursing (international) citations. Also included were four additional citations: (1) a critical review of the study by Gawande and colleagues,[19] (2) one integrated literature review,[20] (3) a discussion of instrument counts extracted from studies,[18] and (4) a review from a statistician's perspective.[21] No studies were conducted as experimental design, but rather retrospective reviews (four medical) of outcomes and a prospective field observation (one medical) of the counting process. The three nursing studies were descriptive studies using questionnaires and interviews. Only one additional citation addressed the process of implementation of evidence-supported recommendations.[22] Most of the remaining citations are general discussions based on reviews of existing studies.

REVIEWING THE EVIDENCE
Study Findings

Retained foreign object events

Three medical studies focused on retained foreign object (RFO) events.[23–25] The variables evaluated fell into three broad categories: (1) patient characteristics, (2) procedure details, and (3) staffing patterns. Patient characteristics included age, gender, and weight. Specific details of the procedure included complexity of the procedure (number of major procedures performed and surgical teams); unplanned changes in procedure; duration of the procedure; emergency status; time of the procedure (eg, off shift, weekend, holiday); body cavity involved; and estimated blood loss. Staffing patterns considered multiple teams involved, change in staff, and the number of circulating nurses and scrub persons per case. **Table 3** summarizes these three studies.

Gawande and colleagues[24] is the most commonly cited study for incidence rate (1:1000–1500). A second study reported a "true" incidence rate (1:5500), described as the number of actual RFOs per total number of procedures. Additionally, 50% of reported cases were actual RFOs and 50% were close calls (near misses).[23] Within these studies, the incidence of retained surgical instruments was as low as 3%[23] up to 31%[24] and 43%,[25] and involved all body cavities. The low percentage reported in the study by Cima and colleagues[23] can be attributed to the institution's protocol for radiographic screening before the patient is transferred to the postanesthesia care unit. With a lack of studies specific to surgical instruments, the true incidence rate is unknown.

Table 3
Summary of published studies on surgical counts and retained foreign object

Study	Research Question	Study Design	Results	Implications
Cima RR et al[23]	What are risk factors and incidence of RFO?	D: retrospective review DB: incident reports of near miss and actual RFO (2003–2006) N: 68 reported cases V: patient characteristics, procedure details, actual RFO data	Rate: 1:5500 N: 68 reports 50% near miss 50% actual RFO 3% instruments Most RFO have correct count documented 59% unexpected detection with standard protocol for radiograph before PACU Risks: breakdown in communication (placement in cavity; failure to remember placement)	True incidence (actual RFO/total number procedures) Discusses near misses Recommended radiograph screening before transfer to PACU
Gawande AA et al[24]	What are risk factors and incidence?	D: retrospective case-control analysis DB: medical malpractice claims and incident reports (1985–2001) N: 54 patients/61 RFOs V: patient characteristics, procedure details, staffing	Rate: 1:1000–1500 N: 54 patients with 69 RFOs Instruments = 31% 88% of RFOs had correct count documented Risk: emergency surgery; higher body mass index, unplanned change in procedure	Widely cited study for incidence and risk factors Provides direction for further study on adjunct strategies
Lincourt AE et al[25]	What are the risk factors associated with RFO after surgery?	D: retrospective case-control analysis DB: cross-referenced procedure code (ICD-9 998.4) with billing/reimbursement data (1996–2005) N: 30 V: patient characteristics; procedure details, staffing, counts performed	Rate: 43% instruments all cavities involved Risk: incorrect counts; multiple major procedures and teams at same time; variables of other studies not significant to this study	Recommended radiograph screening for patients at risk including correct count status

Abbreviations: D, study design; DB, database; N, number; PACU, postanesthesia care unit; RFO, retained foreign object; V, variables.

For risk factors associated with RFO events, Gawande and colleagues[24] is also the most commonly cited study, which identified three significant risk factors: (1) emergency status of the procedure, (2) high body mass index, and (3) unplanned change in surgical procedure. The second study reported communication factors, specifically the failure to communicate to the surgical team members the placement of countable items in the cavity and failure to remember placing the item later on in the procedure.[23] Variables in these studies were not found to be significant in the third study, but rather the outcome of surgical counts as "incorrect" and multiple procedures and teams were found to be significant associated risk factors.[25] The consensus among all three studies was that most RFO events occurred with the count documented as "correct," as high as 88%.[15] Also of note, 59% of the RFOs were detected unexpectedly through postoperative radiograph.[23] **Box 1** summarizes the risk factors. It is interesting to note that in the Teixeira and colleagues[26] study, which focused on RFO events occurring in the high-risk trauma patient population, no retained surgical instruments were reported in the retrospective case review of 2526 cases involving laparotomy, thoracotomy, and sternotomy.

Among countable items there are some differences to consider about surgical instruments. As compared with sponges and sharps, instruments can be taken and returned without passing between the scrub person and surgeon or assistant, are more easily detected and identifiable on imaging, and manifest clinical symptoms in a shorter time frame postoperatively.

Counting process

Two medical and three nursing studies focused on the surgical count process itself.[27–31] The ability of surgical counts to identify and prevent count discrepancies, the rate and type of discrepancies occurring in the counting process, the perceived value of recommended practices for surgical counts, implementation and adherence

---

Box 1
Risk factors associated with RFO

Procedural factors
- Emergency status (nine-time higher risk)
- Unplanned change in procedure (four-time increase)
- Complexity (time or duration, number of procedures and teams)

Patient characteristics
- Higher body mass index

Communication
- Between team members (nurse and surgeon; nurse-nurse and scrub person)
- Placement of item
- Hand-offs

Counts
- Not performed
- "Incorrect" final count (false-negative)

Staffing
- Multiple teams
- Hand-offs

to surgical count protocols, and the communication relationships among the surgical team members (nurse and doctor, nurse-nurse and scrub person) were evaluated. **Table 4** summarizes these studies.

Three studies in particular provide interesting and complementary information about the nuances of the surgical count process.[27,28,31] The ability of counts to detect and prevent an RFO, the types and rate of discrepancies in counts, and the dynamics of the communication relationships among surgical team members were reported. Egorova and colleagues[27] reported a discrepancy rate of 1:7000 or 1 in 70 cases. Surgical counts identified discrepancies in 77% of final counts and prevented 54%. Greenberg and colleagues[28] took the investigation of count discrepancies another level deeper. Observing counting processes in real time within a surgical procedure as compared with aggregate case analysis revealed detailed identification of the type and rate of discrepancies. The results indicated a discrepancy rate of one in eight cases. A per case mean of 16.6 counts requiring 8.6 minutes to perform was reported. Surgical instruments accounted for 34% of the discrepancies. Overall, most discrepancies involved a misplaced item (59%). Documentation errors (38%) and miscounts (3%) accounted for the remaining discrepancies. Risk factors for discrepancies were identified as complexity of the procedure (time or duration of procedure, number of nursing teams) and change in personnel.

Insight into the dynamics of the communication interactions among the surgical team was reported by Riley and colleagues.[31] Counts are performed in a controlled and regulated manner, based on professional recommended practices and institutional policy, including steps for discrepancies. Three major issues were identified that influence the count process: (1) critical judgment, (2) normalization of a routine task, and (3) establishing priorities in complex care environment.

Nurses used professional judgment when there was low risk for a retained item (small incision); relied on each other when there was a question (vs referring to the policy); and "tested" team members' willingness to comply with policy ("do you want another count?"). Another interesting finding was the perception of some colleagues as "sticklers" adhering to policy, whereas others were seen as more flexible.

Counts are a highly regulated practice that can become a routine, taken-for-granted task. Personal and professional ethics can influence the process. Competency and skill level (novice vs experienced) and specialization were noted factors. Specialty teams can recite tray contents by memory; "outsiders" were seen as potentially adding tension when questioning practices that, although they deviated from the policies, had become the normal. Novices whose knowledge of and ability to identify items and who needed more time to perform the surgical count were seen as less competent and efficient by peers and reported a reluctance to acknowledge their needs or challenge questionable practices.

Respondents also reported that it was difficult to conduct counts in the presence of multiple priorities and distractions. Examples cited included the surgeon expecting the scrub person to assist him or her during counting, suspension of counts during emergency or life-threatening situations, and a lack of a procedural pause to conduct surgical counts.

This study indicated that although counting seems to be a straightforward process, complex power relationships and multiple priorities are involved. Counting practices are adapted to the demands of the surgical procedure and influenced by the experience level of the nurses and perceived skill level of team members.

Discussion

Surgical instrument counts are an important patient safety strategy. The available research provides valuable information and understanding in several areas associated

Table 4
Summary of published studies on counting process

Study	Research Question	Study Design	Results	Implications
Egorova NN et al[27]	What is accuracy rate of counts to identify and prevent discrepancies?	D: retrospective review DB: NY State cardiac database; institutional incident reports (2000–2004) N: 1062 count discrepancies V: type of RFO; procedural details	Rate: 1:7000 or 1 in 70 cases with count discrepancy N: final count identified 77% and prevented in 54% Risks: complexity of procedure (time and duration of procedure, multiple nursing teams)	Quantified accuracy of counts to predict and prevent discrepancies and RFOs Discussion provides definitions and clarifications of terminology (true-false positive incorrect counts; true-false negative correct counts)
Greenberg CC et al[28]	What is the rate and type of discrepancies in counts?	D: prospective field observation (individual counting episodes within procedure vs aggregate case) DB: elective general surgery procedures N: 148 procedures V: performance of count protocol, frequency of discrepancies	Rate; 19 cases (12.8%) 1 in 8 cases with count discrepancy 34% instruments 16.6 counting episodes per case (mean) 13 min (average) to resolve discrepancy 8.6 minutes per case 59% misplaced 38% documentation error 3% miscount Risk: incorrect count, change in personnel	

| Riley R et al[31] | How do interactions between nurses and surgeon affect the surgical count in actual practice? | D: Qualitative, ethnographic study with direct field observation and follow-up interviews

DB: 11 operating room nurses in 3 perioperative departments (Melbourne, Australia)

N: 11 operating room nurses per 3 perioperative departments | Count process is highly disciplined and controlled practice as detailed in professional recommended practices and facility policy for variations in counting situations

Forms of power shape and control the practice

Disparities in interpretation and application of policy

Discursive practices affecting surgical count:

a. critical judgment (using professional judgment and skill level of practitioner to meet demands and nature of the procedure)

b. normalization (taken for granted, repetitive routine; deviation becomes new norm)

c. establishing priorities (multiple conflicting priorities) | Mutual commitment to surgical counts as patient safety strategy by all surgical team members

Improve communication skills between surgeons and nurses

Explore innovations in surgical count process |

(continued on next page)

Table 4
(continued)

Study	Research Question	Study Design	Results	Implications
Hamlin L[30]	Does the recommended counting standard prevent retained foreign bodies; what actions are taken for incorrect counts and missing items, including reporting/documentation?	D: ACORN NUM questionnaire DB: perioperative nurse managers; ACORN past and current Board members	85.4% "always" base counting procedure on ACORN Standard; 79% believed that Standard reduced incidence of miscount or RFO; 54% reported miscount in past year with instruments as the third most frequently reported missing item; Method of reporting lost surgical item included incident form, quality activity, direct entry into patient record, report to operating room management committee	Majority opinion that use of ACORN Standard reduces likelihood of incidence of RFO; Need for clarity and consistency within Standard
Ebbeke P[29]	Comparison of theoretical knowledge and clinical practice of surgical counts	D: questionnaire DB: operating rooms nurses attending continuing education activities N: 129 respondents	Facilities define own specific policies versus reference to professional recommended practices R: Written guidelines, 39%, Initial count, 50%, RN count, 92% Documentation,94% Instrument counts documentation,38% Action taken for incorrect count, 99% Surgical count preventing RFO, 64% respondents involved in surgical procedure	Strengths and weaknesses of counting process identified Standard counting process and procedural recommendations for operating room departments to evaluate own policies

Abbreviations: D, study design; DB, database; N, number; RFO, retained foreign object; V, variables.

with surgical counts. Although considered underestimated, a baseline for the rate of incidence of RFO has been quantified. Associated risk factors have been identified in several categories including procedural details (emergency status, complexity, unplanned change in procedure, number of teams involved); patient characteristics (obesity); communication factors dynamics among team members; placement of countable items; hand-offs (breaks, lunch, and change of shift relief); and staffing (number of teams, coordinating hand-offs with counts). Research investigating the count process for accuracy, discrepancies, and real-time counting episodes provides critical insight into the nuances of the counting process.

Recommended practices for manual counting are considered the gold standard. Research reveals vulnerability and susceptibility, however, to human and system factors. Although counting seems to be a simple and routine clinical practice on the surface, it occurs in a complex environment of care with multiple distractions and conflicting priorities. Counts can be time- and labor-intensive, perceived as added workload for the surgical team, and distracting to other patient care needs.[27] Clinicianscan become desensitized to the count process and adapt the counting process to the situation of the procedure, interpreting and adhering to institutional policy based on experience and skill level, both perceived and real. The practice of counting is standard procedure; the process of counting is subject to individualization.[32]

The lack of consistent terminology and standard definitions was discussed in three studies.[21,27,28] The term for RFO varies between studies and investigators (eg, item, object, body, surgical item). The term for a retained sponge is "gossypiboma," but no term has been used in reference to retained surgical instruments.[20] Variations for the definition of RFO in the literature include, "any object unintentionally retained at the time of final wound closure or in procedure without a wound when the operating team has completed the procedure,"[23] and "an item is retained if the patient is no longer in the operating room when an object is found to be inside the patient and a new operation is required to remove it."[17] One study's definition of "retained" refers to a misplaced object located within the patient's body cavity before being transferred from the operating room (a "near miss" or "close call") or postoperatively, then referred to as an "RFO adverse event."[28] The definitions differ as to whether the patient has left the operating room and requires a separate procedure for removal. The Joint Commission and National Quality Forum use the term "retained foreign object." It is important to note that the Joint Commission defines "after surgery" as "any time after completion of the skin closure; even if the patient is still in the OR under anesthesia."[33] The rationale for what seems a stringent definition is based on the premise that it is a significant system failure to not identify and correct an unintentional retention of an object before final wound closure. Future research will produce more comparable rates of incidence by using a standard definition consistent with the Joint Commission.

Selvan and colleagues[21] discussed the conflicting use of "incorrect count." The term has been used regarding errors in the counting process per se (a flaw or error in the counting process) and as the criterion for RFO designation. These authors suggested that the terms "matched" and "unmatched" be used in reference to outcomes of the counting process, indicating agreement or disagreement between initial and final counts. Egorova and colleagues[27] provided four definitions for outcomes of the count process. Correct counts can be false- or true-negatives, and incorrect counts can be true- or false-positives. **Box 2** summarizes suggested terminology. Final counts provide the information that is the most critical for decision making when dealing with the potential for an RFO.

Terminology for any counting problem (discrepancy) when the subsequent count does not agree with the previous count was discussed by Greenberg and

---

Box 2
Terminology used in surgical count processes

Terminology for outcomes of surgical counts

Discrepancy: term used for counting problem; subsequent count does not agree with previous count[28]

Miscount: discrepancy between the number counted and the number actually present; can be undercounted or double counted

Misplaced: unintentional lost item (on floor, in drapes, trash); may or may not be located

Retained item: misplaced item within the patient's body cavity either before or after leaving the operating room

Documentation error: error made in addition; failure to record item

Correct count: agreement between initial and final count

True-negative correct count: no discrepancies and no complications from retained foreign body after 1 year[27]

False-negative correct count: no discrepancies but RFO eventually discovered[27]

Incorrect count: discrepancy between initial and final counts

True-positive incorrect count: count discrepancy and eventual discovery of RFO[27]

False-positive incorrect count: count discrepancy, but missing item not found or located and no complication after 1 year[27]

Matched: initial and final counts agree[21]

Unmatched: initial and final counts do not agree[21]

Terminology for documentation of final counts (refers to the final agreement or disagreement between the initial and final counts)

Correct or matched: no discrepancy encountered or discrepancy reconciled; used only if no RFO event

Incorrect or unmatched: discrepancy that was not reconciled

Terminology for retained foreign object events

"After surgery": any time after completion of the skin closure; even if the patient is still in the operating room under anesthesia[33]

---

colleagues.[28] A "miscount" reflects a difference between the number counted and the number actually present because of a double count or undercount (human error). "Misplaced" refers to unintentional loss in locations, such as trash receptacles and drapes. Misplaced items located in a body cavity are referred to as "retained."

Limitations of Studies

Study design

None of the studies were an experimental, randomized design because it would be unethical to assign patients to a control group that would potentially subject them to harm and adverse outcomes. With case-control analysis, the outcomes of studies are present at the start of the study and conclusions indicate association between risk factors and outcomes rather than causation.[19] The critical review by McCleod and Bohnen[19] of the Gawande and colleagues[24] study cited as limits of the study the small sample size and use of different databases of the two groups, making assessment of comparability between the two difficult.

Database
The use of malpractice and insurance claims and incident report databases may have a selection bias. These may not reflect true incidence, but only those brought into the legal arena as a result of patient harm and resulting compensation.

Nonspecific to instrument counts
The attention to surgical counts as significant to focused patient safety initiatives is relatively recent. No studies exclusive to instruments counts were identified in the literature search; the true incidence of retention of surgical instruments is unknown and the recommendations and conclusions are drawn from the findings of studies of surgical counts in general.

Terminology
A variety of terms with inconsistent definitions are encountered in the literature. Terms for outcomes of counts, documentation of counts, and RFO require clarification and standardization. Variance in terminology and definition may influence patients or cases selected for inclusion in a study sample and results and interpretations.

IMPLICATIONS FOR CLINICAL BEST PRACTICES
Recommendations

Many of the lessons learned from wrong-site surgery research can be applied to surgical instrument counts. Understanding how and why errors occur and the role of human and system factors provides direction in developing counting policies. Administrative support for safe culture, investment in complimentary technology, rapid response teams, and fostering an equal voice for all team members are successful strategies.

Two resources in particular provide detailed discussion and recommendations for prevention of unintentionally RFO. The Institute for Clinical Systems Improvement includes an annotated protocol.[11] The Veterans Health Administration's directive for the Prevention of Retained Surgical Items describes in detail a thorough and methodic wound exploration.[10] Specific recommendations of the literature in this review are provided in **Box 3**.

Emerging Assistive Technology

The consensus in the literature is that multiple systems are needed to complement the manual counting process and verify the final count outcome. Several studies suggested that the technology being used for tracking surgical sponges may be applied to surgical instrumentation. The US Patent Office Web site lists several innovative patent applications for surgical instrument tracking.[34] This emerging technology can potentially be extended to nonradiographic instrumentation items (nonmetallic). The purpose for assistive technology is not to replace the manual counting process, but to provide cognitive reminders to bring attention to the task and provide additional verification methods of the manual counting outcomes. Caution should be taken to not become dependent on technology because it is also subject to human factors and competency and skill in proper and effective application.

IMPLEMENTING EVIDENCE INTO PRACTICE

Most of the literature discusses findings and recommendations, but stops short of offering implementation strategies. One source, however, building on the authors' previous research, described in detail a comprehensive three-phase implementation process: risk analysis, education and training, and evaluation and monitoring.[22]

Box 3
Specific recommendations of the literature

Policies

- Count policy consistent with evidence-based recommended practices
- Standardized counting policy throughout facility
- Counting policy available for reference in each operating room
- Decision tree for count discrepancy events
- Periodic review of policies

Counting aids

- Purposed designed instrument count sheets
    - Specific to each instrument tray
    - Standardized names for instruments, including manufacturer's catalog number
    - Instrument count sheet listed in order of tray assembly
- Evaluate and implement appropriate adjunct and assistive technology

Process

- Consistent adherence to counting protocol
- Limit hand-offs during case, coordinate hand-offs with counts to ensure consistent team for counting process
- Procedural pause for counts ("red rule")[11,22]
- Limit distractions during count process in complex or multiple procedures, second circulator for patient care needs; primary circulator conducts instrument counts
- Count "pieces and parts" (components) of instrumentation separately (eg, wound retractor blades, screws)

Discrepancies

- Decision tree posted and available in each operating room for reference
- Thorough cavity search before closure begins
- Radiographic screening (discrepancy and at-risk patients)
- Imaging request specific for "rule out" retained surgical instrument
    - Name and callback number for surgeon
    - Images read by radiologist
    - Type of surgery
    - Type of instrument missing
- "Parallel process": primary circulator conducts count discrepancy action steps; secondary circulator attends to patient care needs

Competency

- Standardized orientation and training for all members of surgical team (perioperative nurse, scrub technologist, surgeon, medical students, residents), existing staff, new staff as hire on or join facility
- Periodic competency assessment

Self-assessment

The risk analysis can be described as a "know thyself assessment." Examining the incidence of close calls (near misses) and actual retained instruments and the patient population served by the facility for risk (trauma center, obese patient population, and so forth) provides a baseline. Policies and procedures should be reviewed using a set of criteria. Suggested criteria among the studies include

- Current and up to date
- Consistent with evidence-based recommend practices of professional organizations, including terminology
- Standardized throughout the facility or organization in all departments performing surgical and invasive procedures
- Clear description of roles and responsibilities of surgical team members
- Includes protocol for resolution of discrepancies in counts
- Describes documentation of final count outcomes
- Clarifies situations when the count may be omitted or suspended.

The Mayo experience[22] revealed what is probably typical for many facilities: policies amended in response to individual events resulting in protocols that are confusing and difficult to implement.

Education and Training

The purpose of the education and training phase is to deliver a consistent message and performance expectations to the entire surgical team. This includes mandatory education, skills laboratories, and posting of count protocol. Specific steps included an all-staff meeting and extensive educational efforts (morning reports, daily reminders, posting of protocol and quality improvement trends, review of policies, and in-room audits). Improvement of direct communication among team members was stressed in this phase. The education phase included the introduction of a "red rule" for surgical counts. A "red rule" is considered an inviolable rule of conduct in the operating room. All counts must be performed by two team members in the standardized manner. During the closing pause, the surgeon and assistant stop all activity other than the appropriate wound exploration to reduce interruptions to the counting process.

Evaluation and Monitoring

The third phase is evaluation and continuous monitoring. For any patient safety strategy to be successful, consistent adherence to the protocol is vital. Direct observation during actual counting and a rapid response team for near misses (close calls) and actual events are key elements. Critical analysis of a never-event, consistent and periodic feedback to the surgical team on progress toward never-event goals, and addressing cultural and communication issues require administrative involvement, reinforcement, and support for sustained solutions.

Multidisciplinary Team

Achieving patient safety outcomes is becoming increasingly multidisciplinary. The initial step for any implementation strategy is to form a multidisciplinary team. Key stakeholders include perioperative nurses, surgeons, central service staff, radiology staff, risk and quality managers, and administrators. Lessons learned from the clinical pathway and case management experience stress the importance for all members of the surgical team to be at the table to discuss critical elements in the counting protocol. Intraoperative patient safety begins with preoperative preparations. Involving central service staff in the discussion of the importance of consistent instrument tray assembly according to the instrument count sheet as a critical step of the intraoperative counting process reinforces their role and contribution to patient safety. Likewise, radiology staff involved in the development of protocol for imaging verification in the event of discrepancies ensures clear understanding of the needs and expectations for resolution of count discrepancies requiring imaging confirmation.

SUMMARY

With a heightened emphasis on patient safety and a lowered tolerance for the occurrence of never-events there is an obvious need for improved practices. Evidence-based knowledge bridges this gap by providing direction for best practices that ensure consistent and sustained safe patient care and optimal outcomes. Perioperative nursing has a long-standing and well-respected position of advocating for safe patient care. With intimate knowledge of the counting process, perioperative nurses, as key stakeholders in the multidisciplinary approach, must contribute to the body of evidence regarding best practices for effective surgical counts.

REFERENCES

1. AORN. Recommended practices for sponge, sharp, and instrument counts. In: Standards, recommended practices, and guidelines. Denver (CO): AORN, Inc; 2009. p. 405–14.
2. Australian College of Operating Room Nurses. 2008 ACORN standards for perioperative nurses including nursing roles, guidelines, position statements and competency standards. Available at: http://www.acorn.org.au/content/view/60/62/. Accessed June 11, 2009.
3. Australian College of Operating Room Nurses. ACORN count resource package. Available at: http://www.acorn.org.au/content/view/195/122/. Accessed June 11, 2009.
4. Association for Perioperative Practice. Swab, instrument and needle counts: managing the risk. October 2007. Available at: http://www.afpp.org.uk. Accessed June 11, 2009.
5. Operating Room Nurses Association of Canada. Surgical counts in recommended standards, guidelines, and position statements for perioperative nursing practice. Available at: http://www.ornac.ca. Accessed June 12, 2009.
6. South African Theatre Nurses (SATS). Swab, instrument, and needle counts in guidelines for basic theatre procedures. Available at: http://home.mweb.co.za/s./sa.t.s. Accessed June 11, 2009.
7. International Federation of Perioperative Nurses. IFPN guidelines for surgical counts-sponges, sharps, instruments. Available at: http://www.ifpn.org.uk/WebPage.aspx?pageid=23. Accessed June 11, 2009.
8. American College of Surgeons. [ST-51] Statement on the prevention of retained foreign bodies after surgery. Available at: http://www.facs.org/fellows_info/statements/st-51.html. Accessed June 11, 2009.
9. WHO Guidelines for safe surgery First Ed World Alliance for Patient Safety World Health Organization 2008. Available at: http://www.who.int/patientsafety/safesurgery/knowledge_base/WHO_Guidelines_Safe_Surgery_finalJun08.pdf. Accessed June 11, 2009.

10. Department of VA/VHA Directive 2006–030. Prevention of retained surgical items. Available at: http://www1.va.gov/vhapublications/ViewPublication. asp?pub_ID=1425. Accessed June 12, 2009.
11. Institute for Clinical Systems Improvement. Health care protocol: prevention of unintentionally retained foreign objects in surgery. 1st edition, 2007. Available at: http://www.icsi.org/home/retained_foreign_objects_in_surgery__prevention_of_ unintentionally__protocol__21475.html. Accessed June 12, 2009.
12. National Quality Forum. Serious reportable events in healthcare: 2005–2006 update. Available at: http://www.qualityforum.org/projects/completed/sre/. Accessed June 28, 2009.
13. Centers for Medicare and Medicaid. Details for incorporating selected national quality forum and never events into Medicare's list of hospital-acquired conditions. Available at: http://www.cms.hhs.gov/apps/media/press/factsheet-asp? Accessed June 12, 2009.
14. Focus on Five. Preventing retained foreign objects: improving safety after surgery. Joint Comm Perspect Patient Saf 2006;6(3):11.
15. Beyea SC. Counting instruments and sponges. AORN J 2003;78(2):290, 293–4.
16. Standards for sponge, needle, and instrument procedures. AORN J 1976;23(6): 971–3.
17. Gibbs VC. Preventable errors in the operating room: retained foreign bodies after surgery – part 1. Curr Probl Surg 2007;44(6):281–337.
18. Berkowitz S, Marshall H, Charles A. Retained intra-abdominal surgical instruments: time to use nascent technology? Am Surg 2007;73(11):1083–5.
19. McLeod RS, Bohnen JMA. Canadian Association of General Surgeons evidence based reviews in Surgery. 9. Risk factors for retained foreign bodies after surgery. Can J Surg 2004;47(1):57–9.
20. Stawicki SP, Evans DC, Cipolla J, et al. Retained foreign bodies: a comprehensive review of risks and preventive strategies. Scand J Surg 2009;98(1): 8–17.
21. Selvan MS, Skibber JM, Walsh GL. The surgical instrument counting process: a statistician's plea for terminology clarification. J Surg Res 2008;150:1–2.
22. Cima RR, Kollengode A, Storsveen AS, et al. A multidisciplinary team approach to retained foreign objects. Jt Comm J Qual Patient Saf 2009;35(3):123–32.
23. Cima RR, Kollengade A, Garnatz J, et al. Incidence and characteristics of potential and actual retained foreign objects in surgical patients. J Am Coll Surg 2008; 207(1):80–7.
24. Gawande AA, Studdert DM, Orav EJ, et al. Risk factors for retained instruments and sponges after surgery. N Engl J Med 2003;348(3):229–35.
25. Lincourt AE, Harrell A, Cristiano J, et al. Retained foreign bodies after surgery. J Surg Res 2007;138(2):170–4.
26. Teixeira PG, Inaba K, Salim A, et al. Retained foreign bodies after emergent trauma surgery: incidence after 2526 cavitary explorations. Am Surg 2007; 73(10):1031–4.
27. Egorova NN, Moskowitz A, Gelijns A, et al. Managing the prevention of retained surgical instruments: what is the value of counting? Ann Surg 2008;247(1): 13–8.
28. Greenberg CC, Regenbogen SE, Lipsitz SR, et al. The frequency and significance of discrepancies in the surgical count. Ann Surg 2008;248(2):337–41.
29. Ebbeke P. [Retained foreign bodies from the view of the OR nurse]. Chirurg 2007; 78(1):13–21.

30. Hamlin L. Setting the standard: the role of ACORN. Part II: counting, the gold standard to prevent the inadvertent retention of surgical items or is it? ACORN Winter, 2006;19(2):24–5.
31. Riley R, Manias E, Polglase A. Governing the surgical count through communication interactions: implications for patient safety. Qual Saf Health Care 2006;15(5): 369–74.
32. Gibbs VC. Patient safety practices in the operating room: correct-site surgery and no thing left behind. Surg Clin North Am 2005;85(6):1307–19.
33. The Joint Commission. FAQ: retained foreign object after surgery. Available at: http://www.jointcommission.org/NR/rdonlyres/6215419C-2DEA-41F4-B91D-FF119C006048/0/retained_foreign_objects_faqs.pdf. Accessed May 22, 2009.
34. US Patent Office. Available at: http://uspto.gov. Accessed June 21, 2009.

The Hands-Free Technique: An Effective and Easily Implemented Work Practice

Bernadette Stringer, PhD[a,b],*, Theodore Haines, MD, MSc[c]

KEYWORDS
• Work practice • Hands-free technique • Blood-borne

A series of prospective United States operating room studies published between 1990 and 2002, in which dedicated observers or circulating nurses recorded blood and body-fluid exposures, found that percutaneous injuries occurred in 1.1% to 15% of all surgeries, and mucocutaneous contaminations occurred in 1.4% to 32.1% of all surgeries.[1–7] In these studies, surgeons and residents usually sustained the greatest number of percutaneous and other exposures during surgery. However, in one operating room study, scrubbed personnel sustained as many percutaneous injuries as surgeons[2] and, in another, circulating nurses sustained the greatest total number of contaminations, although surgeons sustained the greatest number of percutaneous injuries.[6] Two of these studies, in addition to measuring occupational exposures, also measured patient wound recontact rates. One study found a patient wound recontact rate of 32%, and the other found a patient wound recontact rate of 11%.[5,6]

Since these studies were conducted, operating room risk has not decreased, according to blood and body-fluid exposure surveillance data from 87 United States hospitals participating in the Exposure Prevention Information Network (EPINet). More specifically, after passage of the US Needlestick Safety and Prevention Act in 2000, which strengthened the requirement to use reengineered sharp safety devices, percutaneous injuries decreased by 34% from 2000 to 2004 in hospital departments

[a] Occupational Health and Safety Agency for Healthcare in BC (OHSAH), Suite 301 - 1195 West Broadway, Vancouver, BC V6H 3X5, Canada
[b] Faculty of Health Sciences, Simon Fraser University, Burnaby, BC, Canada
[c] Department of Clinical Epidemiology and Biostatistics, Faculty of Health Sciences, Health Sciences Centre, McMaster University, Room 3H54, 1200 Main Street West, Hamilton, ON L8N 3Z5, Canada
* Corresponding author. Occupational Health and Safety Agency for Healthcare in BC (OHSAH), Suite 301 - 1195 West Broadway, Vancouver, BC V6H 3X5, Canada.
E-mail addresses: bernadettes@ohsah.bc.ca; bstringer@shaw.ca

Perioperative Nursing Clinics 5 (2010) 45–58
doi:10.1016/j.cpen.2009.11.002
1556-7931/10/$ – see front matter © 2010 Elsevier Inc. All rights reserved.

periopnursing.theclinics.com

outside the operating room, but they remained relatively unchanged in the operating room.[8] As a result, the proportion of all hospital percutaneous injuries occurring in the operating room has risen steadily from 25% in 2000 to 35.2% in 2006.[9] The reason that the operating room injury rates have held almost steady, even though rates outside the operating room have fallen, has been attributed primarily to underuse of reengineered sharp safety devices, such as blunt suture needles and safety scalpels. Weak compliance with double gloving and hands-free passing also likely have contributed to maintaining these stubborn injury rates in the operating room.[10]

This ongoing risk exists within the context of widespread underreporting of occupational exposures by all surgical personnel and of low hepatitis B immunization rates among surgeons. Underreporting varies by occupational group,[11] although it continues to be highest among surgeons[12,13] and surgical residents.[14] In a recent national study in the United States, for example, 51% of 699 surgical residents surveyed had not reported their most recent percutaneous injury to employee health, including 16% with high-risk injuries.[14] Most salaried personnel and surgical trainees have complied with hepatitis B immunization since the 1980s, but this is not necessarily the case for surgeons. For example, a recent survey of United States transplant surgeons found that 23% of 311 respondents had not received the required number of doses of the hepatitis B vaccine to guarantee immunity.[15]

This article reviews the evidence on the effectiveness of hands-free passing, one of the safety measures recommended to decrease blood-borne exposure risk.

THE HANDS-FREE TECHNIQUE

Implementation of the hands-free technique to reduce blood-borne exposure risk during surgery was first recommended by the Association of periOperative Registered Nurses (AORN) in the early 1990s.[16] Since then, other professional nursing and surgical organizations[17,18] have also recommended its use as has the Occupational Safety and Health Administration (OSHA).[19] Specifically, in a 2007 Standard Interpretations letter, one of several OSHA letters on this topic, the director stated, "Hospitals must implement the use of...proper work practices, such as designated neutral or safe zones, which allow hands-free passing of sharps."[20] OSHA also highlights hands-free passing on its hospital e-tool, Surgical Suite Module.[21]

The hands-free technique is a work practice whereby no two members of the surgical team handle the same sharp item at the same time. When the hands-free technique is implemented, sharp items are not passed hand to hand between surgeons, residents, scrub personnel, and circulating personnel. Instead, sharp items are laid down in one or more designated "neutral" zones for retrieval, where they are returned during or after use.

Sharp items referred to consist of suture needles, scalpels, trocars, and any other items that can perforate the skin or gloves. Neutral zones can be implemented by using receptacles already in routine use, such as rectangular trays, Mayo stands, or sections of the surgical field, or by specially purchased disposable containers or plastic or magnetic drapes. Sharp items should fit comfortably within receptacles or on tables selected as neutral zones. Whether one or more neutral zone is established during surgery, and where zones are located, should be decided case by case. This depends on the type of surgery, the number of sharp items expected to be used, and the number of personnel working near the surgical wound (**Fig. 1**).

The hands-free technique requires coordination among scrub nurses or technologists, surgeons, residents, and physician assistants and therefore affects the surgical team as a whole. This is why the synchronized performance of the team as a whole

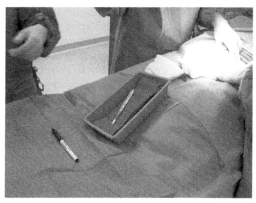

Fig. 1. Hands-free passing using a rectangular tray. (*Courtesy of* Dr William Schecter.)

forms the basis for an accurate estimate of the use of the hands-free technique during surgeries. For example, when the hands-free technique is used most of the time during surgical cases, nurses and scrub personnel lay most or all sharp items onto a neutral zone for retrieval by surgeons and residents. After retrieving and using the instruments, the surgeons and residents lay them or drop them onto a neutral zone for retrieval by scrub personnel. Regardless of whether the hands-free technique is used to exchange a few or many instruments, the interdependence between scrub personnel and surgeons and residents remains fundamental and is why estimates about use of the hands-free technique cannot rely only on assessments of individual use, as was erroneously done in one study.[5]

Increasing Predictability During Surgery

Many aspects of surgery, because of their complexity, do not lend themselves to greater standardization. However, greater standardization can be applied to the routine transferring of sharp items.[22] The hands-free technique streamlines transfers and should increase predictability so that surgical personnel can better anticipate how sharp items will be transferred among them. This is important because surgeons, residents, nurses, and others, as they pass sharp items to each other, will on occasion become distracted, misunderstand requests, or lose control of instruments. Injuries and even deaths can result. In one incident, a scrub nurse sustained a percutaneous injury as a cardiac surgeon tried to return a scalpel to her while she was passing an instrument to another surgeon.[23] In the second incident, a circulating nurse sustained a needlestick as a surgeon passed her an uncapped syringe filled with blood to be sent for hepatitis C testing. That nurse contracted the disease and died a few months later.[24]

Receiving sharp items appears to create the greatest risk. When an individual passes a sharp item, he or she is more likely than the recipient to recognize the risk and act with caution. The intended recipient, however, may not be as actively engaged in what is occurring. Of course this varies. It may be that a surgeon has requested a sharp item and has stopped activity while waiting for it, or that, after giving verbal notification, a scrub nurse waits to pass a sharp item until it is obvious that the surgeon is ready to receive it. But this is frequently not what transpires; therefore, laying sharp items down for retrieval is likely to decrease the level of vigilance required. For example, while scrub personnel are asked to remember to announce that sharp items are being passed, failure to take this precaution becomes less important during hands-free passing. Hands-free passes may also save time because there is not the need to ensure that sharp items are correctly and securely placed in recipients' hands.

The nature of surgical teams and their work represents another reason for increasing predictability. Surgical teams are made up of diverse professionals who may or may not regularly work together and who carry out complex tasks, often under pressure. For example, in a recent study, it was found that 50% of operating room nurses in six Canadian hospitals did not identify themselves as belonging to a specific surgical subspecialty because they "rotated" among three to four specialties on a permanent basis.[25] As well, operating room personnel wear caps, surgical masks, face shields or goggles, and surgical gowns, making it more difficult to communicate. Therefore words are more likely to be muffled and gestures that could enhance the meaning of words in everyday life may not be possible to use. Also, there is growing evidence that operating rooms are noisy, further interfering with good communication during surgery.[26]

DOES THE HANDS-FREE TECHNIQUE REDUCE RISK?

Four studies published between 1997 and 2009 have evaluated the hands-free technique's ability to reduce the risk of percutaneous injuries, glove tears, and mucocutaneous contamination during surgery; three were positive[7,27,28] and one was negative.[29] The following section describes the methods, results, and most important potential limitations of each study.

Eggleston and Colleagues, 1997

A 1997 study by Eggleston and colleagues[29] did not find that using the hands-free technique reduced glove tears during cesarean births. In this randomized controlled trial, consecutive cesarean births during a given interval were individually randomized to receive the intervention or to be control surgeries. During intervention surgeries, personnel were to pass all scalpels, suture needles, and electrocautery tips in trays, and a Mayo stand was to be placed between surgeons, assistants, and scrub technicians for them to also use a neutral zone if they desired. During control surgeries, personnel were to carry on their usual practice. At the end of each case, all gloves worn by surgeons, assistants, and technicians were to be tested for punctures. In addition, all surgical personnel present during a case (intervention or control surgeries) were asked to record information about their role on the surgical team, level of experience, dominant hand, and whether or not they had observed a glove tear during the surgery.

Rates of glove perforation during intervention and control surgeries were then compared. The total number of cesarean births eligible for the study during the study period was 192, of which 165 were randomized to be intervention or control surgeries; of the 165 surgeries, 9 were excluded because none of the personnel saved gloves or recorded required data. In the remaining 156 included surgeries, the rate of glove perforations was 19% in intervention surgeries and 16.1% in control surgeries. This was not a statistically significant difference ($P = .5$).

Potential limitations

Usually, the best design to use in clinical intervention studies is a randomized control trial. However, in this study, such a design introduced a critical limitation because randomization was at the level of the surgery. This meant that, in surgeries selected as intervention surgeries, surgical personnel had to altogether change their usual practice during that case. If the next randomized surgery was a control surgery, then the same surgical team had to return to their usual practice. It is difficult for personnel to change their practice case by case. Changing methods from one case to the next increased the likelihood that one method or the other was not strictly followed. That is, hands-free passing may not have been wholly implemented during intervention surgeries, and hands-free passing may not have been wholly avoided during control surgeries. This issue is especially problematic in this study because there was no independent assessment made about the rate of hands-free passing in a sample of both intervention and control surgeries.

A randomized design could have been used if randomization had been performed at the cluster level (ie, at the level of the hospital). In such a trial, operating room personnel in intervention hospitals would have used hands-free passing in all surgeries and operating room personnel in control hospitals would have continued to practice as usual.

The other serious limitation is that 444 pairs of gloves were tested for punctures when it was reported that 596 personnel were involved in the 156 cesarean births included in the study. Nothing is mentioned about why no testing was done on at least 152 pairs of gloves (perhaps more [some personnel may have worn more than one pair]). The status of the untested gloves could have radically altered the perforation rate comparisons that were made.

This study also had other methodological problems. For example, reasons were not given why 14% of eligible surgeries were not randomized when they should have been. This problem in combination with the problem of randomization and the failure to test a large number of gloves make this study of little use for assessing the effectiveness of hands-free passing.

Folin and Colleagues, 2000

The pretest/posttest design study performed by Folin and colleagues[27] found that hands-free passing decreased percutaneous injuries and contaminations. This study was conducted in a large Swedish university hospital in which data were collected in 357 orthopedic surgeries over 6 weeks preintervention, and in 383 orthopedic surgeries over 6 weeks postintervention; between periods, a 2-week intervention was implemented that consisted of training surgical personnel to use hands-free passing and to manipulate sharp instruments with other instruments instead of fingers (eg, using forceps to load needle drivers). Also, certain sharp surgical instruments were blunted.

Data collection during both study periods was performed by scrub personnel who completed a questionnaire at the end of each surgery asking details about the procedure, the number of personnel involved, and whether a contamination or percutaneous injury had occurred. In surgeries in which exposures occurred, the persons involved completed preintervention and postintervention questionnaires providing details about the incident. Those completing these questionnaires postintervention were also asked to provide information about using the hands-free technique and instruments to manipulate sharps. Incident rates were compared using Fisher's exact tests.

In total, 13 injuries and 11 contaminations occurred in the 357 baseline surgeries, and 6 injuries and 4 contaminations occurred in 383 postintervention surgeries. The decrease in incidents postintervention compared to preintervention was statistically significant ($P<.05$). When examined by occupation, it was found that scrub personnel had a significantly reduced number of injuries postintervention (0 injuries) compared to those occurring preintervention (6 injuries).

Potential limitations

In this study, three separate measures were simultaneously introduced after a baseline period: the hands-free technique, manipulation of sharp items with instruments instead of fingers, and the blunting of certain instruments. Penetration of the interventions was not assessed postintervention. The only information on hands-free technique use collected was after persons were injured or contaminated. Because the degree of uptake of these interventions was not independently assessed, it is not possible to distinguish, let alone speculate about, their separate effects on injury or contamination rates.

For feasibility reasons, this study also had to rely on scrub personnel to provide information for each case once it was completed, and on injured or contaminated personnel to provide details related to their exposures. Because an independent assessment of the data provided by scrub nurses and exposed personnel was not made, it is difficult to assess data quality. Analyses in this study were simple comparisons of proportions of all incidents postintervention compared with preintervention, and then percutaneous injuries and contamination were compared by occupational group. In neither this study nor that of Eggleston and colleagues were statistics adjusted to take into account potential confounding factors, such as length of procedures or degree of blood loss.

Stringer and Colleagues, 2002

This prospective cohort study by Stringer and colleagues[7] found that use of the hands-free technique 75% or more of the time in surgery reduced the risk of percutaneous injuries, glove tears, and contaminations in surgeries in which 100 mL or more of blood loss occurred. This United States study included 3765 surgeries of all types and duration, performed in a large inner-city hospital, where use of the hands-free technique was policy.

In this study, trained circulating and scrub nurses jointly estimated hands-free technique use by the surgical team as a whole at the end of each surgery. Estimates were each assigned one of five categories: about 0%, about 25%, about 50%, about 75%, and about 100%. Circulating nurses also recorded on a questionnaire the length, type, and emergency status of the surgery; amount of blood loss; and number of people present 75% or more of the time (factors that have been associated with increased risk in other studies). In surgeries in which percutaneous injuries, glove tears, and mucocutaneous contaminations occurred, circulators also recorded details of incidents as soon as possible after they occurred.

For quality-control purposes (ie, to determine whether nurses' estimates of hands-free technique use by the surgical team as a whole were accurate), an independent assessment was also performed in 68 surgeries, and the estimated kappa was found to be 0.72 (95% CI 0.54–0.90), indicating "substantial agreement."[30]

Based on a 70% response rate (3765 out of 5388 eligible surgeries), this study found that use of the hands-free technique about 75% or more of the time occurred in 42% of all surgeries. Using logistic regression to adjust for other potential risk factors simultaneously, Stringer and colleagues found that when the hands-free technique was used 75% or more of the time compared with when the hands-free technique was used 50% or less, there were 59% (odds ratio 0.41 [95% CI 0.23–0.72]) fewer percutaneous injuries, glove tears, and contaminations in surgeries in which 100 mL or more blood loss occurred.

Potential limitations

The potential problem with this study is its dependence on circulating and scrub nurses to make estimates on the use of the hands-free technique and on circulators to gather other data. To address this, measures were put in place to track the reliability of estimates and encourage rigorous and accurate collection of data. For example, to encourage nurses to fully complete questionnaires and to prompt eligible surgical personnel to report their injuries, tears, and contaminations and to provide details as soon as possible, weekly raffles for prizes and other incentives were used. To make sure that the hands-free technique use was accurately quantified, circulating nurses consulted with scrub personnel at the end of each surgical case to arrive at estimates. This was done so that personnel most involved in the transfer of sharps were also involved in deriving estimates. In addition, to ensure the accuracy of hands-free technique use estimates, an independent observer also quantified the use of the hands-free technique in a sample of 68 surgeries for comparison to estimates made by circulating and scrub nurses in the same surgeries, resulting in a highly reliable estimate (kappa statistic).

This study also addressed another possible limitation: potential confounding by risk factors independently associated with increased risk of injury, contamination, and glove tear in previous studies (ie, length, type, and emergency status of the surgery; number of personnel present during the surgery; time of day; and blood loss). The study took these potential confounders into account through a statistical method of analysis called *unconditional logistic regression* to enable the simultaneous adjustment of the different risk profiles of surgeries, in which the hands-free technique was used 75% or more of the time and in which the hands-free technique was used 50% or less of the time. This statistical method was not applied in either of the previous studies assessing the hands-free technique's ability to reduce risk.

Stringer and Colleagues, 2009

A 2009 preintervention and postintervention study by Stringer and colleagues[28] found that use of the hands-free technique 75% or more of the time in surgery reduced the risk of percutaneous injuries, glove tears, and contaminations in all types of surgery. Before the preintervention and postintervention study, a qualitative study, in which 20 semistructured telephone interviews were performed with United States and Canadian operating room nurses and surgeons, was conducted to elaborate on reasons why personnel used or did not use the hands-free technique and to formulate suggestions on overcoming barriers to hands-free technique use.[31] Once completed, information from the interviews, previous knowledge about the hands-free technique, technical guidance, and adult education principles were combined to produce an educational video/DVD encouraging proper use of the hands-free technique during different types of surgery. The newly developed hands-free technique video/DVD, titled "Passing Sharps Safely: The Hands-Free Technique," was used as the main component of the intervention implemented during the study.

The study took place in six hospitals in three Canadian cities; three hospitals were control sites and three were intervention sites. At the start of the study, control hospitals had a policy in place recommending use of the hands-free technique. Policies were introduced in two of the intervention hospitals during the study. One intervention hospital did not have a policy in place at the end of the study. Data were collected during three periods in intervention hospitals (baseline and postintervention periods 3 to 4 months apart) and during four periods in control hospitals (three nonintervention periods followed by an intervention period). In intervention hospitals, data were collected during baseline period 1. Then the hands-free technique video/DVD was shown over the course of a week until the commencement of period 2. Then data were collected again during period 3, more than 3 months later. In control hospitals, data were also collected during three periods. Then, after data collection was complete in period 3, the hands-free technique video/DVD was shown for 1 week followed by data collection during period 4 (**Fig. 2**).

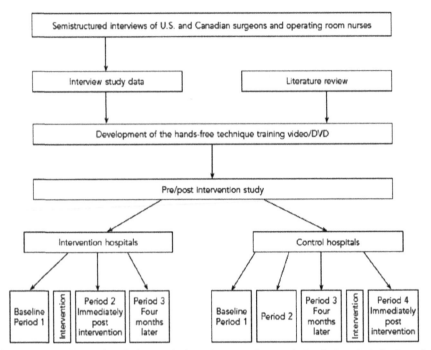

Fig. 2. Pre– and post–hands-free technique intervention study in six hospitals in Canada. (*From* Stringer B, Haines T, Goldsmith CH, et al. Hands-free technique in the operating room: reduction in body fluid exposure and the value of a training video. Public Health Rep 2009;124(Suppl 1):169–79; with permission.)

Data collection methods in this study were similar to those used in the 2002 study by Stringer and colleagues. The hands-free technique use was estimated by circulating nurses and scrub personnel together. At the end of each surgery, circulating nurses recorded information on hands-free technique use and on the same other potential risk factors addressed in the 2002 study. Circulating nurses also recorded details on percutaneous injuries, glove tears, and mucocutaneous contaminations in surgeries when they occurred. To ensure that estimates of hands-free technique use were accurate, independent observers also estimated hands-free technique use in a subset of 30 operations in which the observation time was 75% or more of the surgery's duration. When nurses' and observers' hands-free technique use estimates were compared, the estimated kappa was 0.88 (95% CI 0.80–0.96), considered "almost perfect agreement."[30]

Based on a 60.7% response rate (10,596 of 17,461 eligible surgeries), this study found that use of the hands-free technique about 75% or more of the time occurred in 35% of all surgeries. When unconditional logistic regression was used to adjust for other potential risk factors simultaneously, it was found that when the hands-free technique was used 75% or more of the time, compared with use 50% or less of the time, there were 35% (odds ratio 0.65 [95% CI 0.43–0.97]) fewer percutaneous injuries, glove tears, and contaminations in all types surgeries regardless of blood loss.

This study also found that the newly developed hands-free technique training video shown during intervention sessions increased hands-free technique use to about 75% or more of the time immediately after the intervention, and that increases were sustained for at least 5 months. While there was an overall tendency to increased hands-free technique use in all hospitals during the study, the increase was statistically significantly greater in intervention hospitals compared with control hospitals.

Specifically, 75% to 100% hands-free technique use rates at the control hospitals increased from 24.1% to 32.2% between baseline period 1 and period 2, but this was a smaller increase than at the intervention hospitals. At one intervention hospital, the increase went from 2.6% to 27.7%, and at the other two intervention hospitals it went from an average rate of 10.6% to 22.7%. When hands-free technique use of 75% to 100% was compared between period 3 and period 2, it was found to have increased minimally in the control hospitals, that it was not sustained 5 months later in one intervention hospital where it had fallen from 27.7% in period 2 to 10.7% in period 3 (this was still significantly higher than at baseline when it was 2.6%), and that in the remaining intervention hospital (the other intervention hospital had dropped out of the study), hands-free technique use of 75% to 100% had gone from 24.9% in period 2 to 44.1% in period 3 (5 months later).

Investigators also found that increased use of the hands-free technique may have occurred for another unexpected reason: A policy recommending use was in place or was being considered. In the intervention hospital where a hands-free technique policy was implemented after period 2 and data were collected during period 3, use of the hands-free technique 75% or more of the time in surgery increased by 19%, while in the intervention hospital, where there was no intention of putting a policy in place, hands-free technique use of 75% or more decreased by 14%, although it remained higher than it was preintervention. Use of the hands-free technique 75% or more of the time in surgery occurred in 43% of baseline surgeries in the control hospitals where a hands-free technique policy had been in place for 5 years, and in 11% of baseline surgeries in the two intervention hospitals where a hands-free technique policy was being formulated. Meanwhile, in the other intervention hospital, where a policy was not being considered and is still not in place today, increased hands-free technique use occurred in approximately 3% of baseline surgeries. This means that, although use of the hands-free technique about 75% or more of the time during surgery occurred in 35% of all surgeries included in this study, it occurred in 48% of all surgeries performed in hospitals that had a hands-free technique policy at the start of the study or that implemented a policy during the study.

Potential limitations
This study had the same potential limitation as the previous study by Stringer and colleagues: reliance on information collected by nurses on risk factors, hands-free technique use, and details of incidents as they occurred. Similar measures were applied to address this limitation. For example, incentives were offered to promote the collection of accurate data and a reliability study was conducted to ensure that hands-free technique use estimates were accurate.

However, unlike in Stringer and colleagues' 2002 study, this study missed blood loss data for 27% of surgeries. To address this, multiple imputation (a statistical technique recognized for generating valid inferences for missing data, while reducing the risk of biased results and increasing study power) was used with confidence because of the large number of surgeries included in this study.[32] Missing data were not a problem for other variables.

Before performing the main regression analyses in this study, investigators examined initial assessments of the patterns in hands-free technique use and incidents during each data collection period potentially suggestive of a Hawthorne effect. Surgeries in each period were grouped into fifths by date, and regressions were done for each period to determine if the "fifths" were related to hands-free technique use or incident rates, controlling for type of surgery and hospital. Analyses revealed no indication that surgeries at the beginning of each period were associated with higher reported hands-free technique use and, although they suggested that incident rates were higher in the first fifth of period 1 only, cross-tabulation showed that they were higher in only two of the six study hospitals, which suggested no consistent Hawthorne effect on the study overall.

As in the first study by Stringer and colleagues, potential confounding was addressed using logistic regression as described above.

RATES OF HANDS-FREE PASSING

Implementing hands-free passing is inexpensive, requires little training, and does not appear to have adverse effects. Even so, Stringer and colleagues[7,28] found that in only 42% of surgeries in one study and 35% of surgeries in a second study did surgical teams use the hands-free technique 75% or more of the time. Results from these studies were based on hands-free technique use estimates made at the end of 3765 and 10,596 surgeries, respectively, by circulating nurses and scrub personnel.

Information is available on hands-free technique use in other countries, although this information is based on self-reports collected in surveys. In one study, a national survey of Australian operating room nurses, it was found that 72% of participants "always pass sharps using the hands-free technique."[33] In another study, a survey of operating room nurses in seven hospitals in the Republic of Korea, it was found that 2% always used the hands-free technique and 8% used it most of the time.[34] Hands-free technique use by surgical teams in sufficiently large samples of surgeries should be assessed more broadly and should not rely on self-reports because these are often inflated, as may have occurred in the Australian study.[33]

The findings in the most recent study by Stringer and colleagues—that the overall rate of hands-free technique use of 75% or more of the time was found in only 35% of Canadian surgeries—is especially alarming for two reasons: (1) because this estimate is based on preintervention and postintervention surgeries and (2) because this study took place a decade later than the previous United States study by Stringer and colleagues, which found that hands-free technique use of 75% or more occurred in 42% of surgeries. The relatively low levels of hands-free passing in Canada probably reflects weaker rules because none of its provinces have regulations comparable to the US Bloodborne Pathogens Standard.

INCREASING HANDS-FREE TECHNIQUE USE

The hands-free technique video/DVD developed by Stringer and colleagues[28] is recommended to increase compliance. A shortened version of it has been developed and can be freely accessed (http://www.healthsystem.virginia.edu/Internet/safetycenter/internetsafetycenterwebpages/SafetyinSurgery/SafetyinSurgery.cfm).

In addition, based on Stringer and colleagues' most recent study, it is also reasonable to recommend the development of a comprehensive hands-free technique policy for hospital operating rooms. Such a policy should include a statement recommending use, the definition of the technique, how neutral zones can be arranged, and which items are considered sharp. A policy could also refer to OSHA statements on hands-free technique use found in the legislation or in Standard Interpretation letters.[20]

Evidence on the importance of hands-free technique training can also be found in another preintervention and postintervention study that implemented training and goal setting. This study found that the percentage of sharp instruments passed hands-free increased from 32% to 64% in the inpatient operating room and from 31% to 70% in the outpatient operating room.[35] Meanwhile, the qualitative study conducted before development of the hands-free technique video/DVD for Stringer and colleagues' 2009 study[31] has also provided insights on training and other related issues and on hands-free technique use. More specifically, surgeons who were more resistant to using the hands-free technique than operating room nurses provided fewer suggestions about ways to increase use of the hands-free technique and emphasized that they did not use it because there was a lack of evidence demonstrating the hands-free technique's effectiveness. However, surgeons who underscored this lack of evidence about the hands-free technique's effectiveness did not consistently wear two pairs of gloves during surgery or use blunt suture needles—risk-reduction measures that have been demonstrated to reduce the risk of percutaneous injuries in repeated, rigorously performed studies.[36–38] Nevertheless, this qualitative study also identified that the lack of hands-free technique training among nurses may represent another important barrier to wider use of the technique. The surgeons stated that their resistance would likely decrease if nurses were trained and could adapt hands-free technique use to a variety of procedures. An example of the type of flexibility that training could provide was given by one of the operating room nurses interviewed in the study: "The surgeon needed space on the Mayo stand for all his instruments, and he liked the scalpel up there all the time, so...I used a smaller dish and kept it up there all the time....I handed him the dish with my hand underneath the dish so that he could reach it." Another barrier, identified by both surgeons and operating room nurses, was shift of gaze from the surgical site or from a microscope when retrieving or returning sharps to or from a neutral zone. This potential barrier requires clarification since it is important not to make the error of equating shift of gaze from a surgical site to removing eyes from a microscope. This is because a gaze can usually be shifted without losing procedural continuity, and thus learning to shift one's gaze should be seen as no more than acquiring a new surgical skill.

Although it is hoped that barriers such as those mentioned above can be overcome, it is also important to remember that OSHA enforcement is another tool that can be used to increase hands-free passing. As mentioned in the introduction, the overall percutaneous injury rate in hospital departments outside the operating room had decreased by 34% during the 4-year period after passage of The Needlestick Safety and Prevention Act in 2000. During that same period, the number of hospital citations issued by OSHA under the Bloodborne Pathogens Standard for failure to use engineering and work practice controls, was four times greater than in the previous decade.[8] This appears to mean that OSHA's citations primarily targeted patient areas outside the operating room and suggests that, if the operating room received the same level of attention, there would also be a decline in its percutaneous injury rates.

SUMMARY

The blood and body-fluid exposure risk of operating room personnel and, to a lesser extent, their patients, is ongoing, and use of the hands-free technique and other effective measures should be implemented during surgery, especially because hands-free passing can be done easily and inexpensively. Compliance with use of the hands-free technique can be achieved using a variety of measures; most important, though, is sound educational information on its use, such as that available from viewing the video/DVD accessible on the Internet demonstrating appropriate use in a variety of surgeries.

REFERENCES

1. Gerberding JL, Littell C, Tarkington A, et al. Risk of exposure of surgical personnel to patients' blood during surgery at San Francisco General Hospital. N Engl J Med 1990;322(25):1788–93.
2. Panlilio AL, Foy DR, Edwards JR, et al. Blood contacts during surgical procedures. JAMA 1991;265(12):1533–7.
3. Popejoy SL, Fry DE. Blood contact and exposure in the operating room. Surg Gynecol Obstet 1991;172(6):480–3.
4. Quebbeman EJ, Telford GL, Hubbard S, et al. Risk of blood contamination and injury to operating room personnel. Ann Surg 1991;214(5):614–20.
5. Tokars JI, Bell DM, Culver DH, et al. Percutaneous injuries during surgical procedures. JAMA 1992;267(21):2899–904.
6. White MC, Lynch P. Blood contact and exposures among operating room personnel: a multicenter study. Am J Infect Control 1993;21(5):243–8.
7. Stringer B, Infante-Rivard C, Hanley J. Effectiveness of the hands-free technique in reducing operating theatre injuries. Occ Env Med 2002;59(10):703–7. Available at: http://www.pubmedcentral.nih.gov/articlerender.fcgi?artid=1740223. Accessed June 27, 2009.
8. Jagger J, Perry J, Gomaa A, et al. The impact of U.S. policies to protect healthcare workers from bloodborne pathogens: the critical role of safety-engineered devices. J Infect Public Health 2008;1(2):62–71.
9. International Healthcare Worker Safety Center, University of Virginia. U.S. Epinet needlestick and sharps injury surveillance network. Sharps injury data report for 2000 (26 hospitals contributing 1,787 PI) and 2006 (33 hospitals contributing 950 PI) total injuries. Available at: http://www.healthsystem.virginia.edu/internet/epinet/epinetdatareports.cfm#reports. Accessed June 27, 2009.
10. Dagi TF, Berguer R, Moore S, et al. Preventable errors in the operating room—part 2: retained foreign objects, sharps injuries, and wrong site surgery. Curr Probl Surg 2007;44(6):352–81.
11. Doebbeling BN, Vaughn TE, McCoy KD, et al. Percutaneous injury, blood exposure, and adherence to standard precautions: Are hospital-based health care providers still at risk? Clin Infect Dis 2003;37(8):1006–13.
12. Au E, Gossage JA, Bailey SR. The reporting of needlestick injuries sustained in theatre by surgeons: are we under-reporting? J Hosp Infect 2008;70(1):66–70.
13. Thomas WJ, Murray JR. The incidence and reporting rates of needle-stick injury amongst UK surgeons. Ann R Coll Surg Engl 2009;91(1):12–7.
14. Makary MA, Al-Attar Ali, Holzmueller CG, et al. Needlestick injuries among surgeons in training. N Engl J Med 2007;356(26):2693–9.
15. Halpern SD, Asch DA, Shaked A, et al. Inadequate hepatitis B vaccination and post-exposure evaluation among transplant surgeons. Ann Surg 2006;244(2):305–9.
16. Association of Perioperative Registered Nurses. Recommended practices for standard and transmission-based precautions in the perioperative practice setting. Standards, recommended practices and guidelines. Denver (CO): AORN Inc; 2005. 615–9.
17. American College of Surgeons. Statement on sharps safety [ST-58]. Available at: http://www.facs.org/fellows_info/statements/st-58.html. Accessed June 27, 2009.

18. Operating Room Nurses Association of Canada. "Module 3: Safety/risk prevention and management," in recommended standards, guidelines and position statements for perioperative nursing. 6th edition. Mississauga (ON): Canadian Standards Association; 2006. p. 1–88.

19. Occupational Safety and Health Administration (OSHA). Occupational exposure to blood borne pathogens; needlesticks and other sharps injuries: final rule. 29 CFR 1910.1030. Fed Reg 2001;66:5318–25.

20. Fairfax RE, Directorate of enforcement programs. Letter to Eric Frederik, Director of Safety, Baptist Medical Center. San Antonio 2007 January 17. Available at: http://www.osha.gov/pls/oshaweb/owadisp.show_document?p_table= INTERPRETATIONS&p_id=25620. Accessed June 27, 2009.

21. Stringer B, Infante-Rivard C, Hanley J. The effectiveness of the hands-free technique in reducing operating room injuries. NIOSH's Best practices in workplace surveillance, Cincinnati (OH) November 7–9, 2001. Available at (Hospital e tool, Surgical Suite Module, Bloodborne pathogens): http://www.osha.gov/SLTC/etools/hospital/surgical/surgical.html#BloodbornePathogens. Accessed June 27, 2009.

22. Grote G, Zala-Mezö E. The effects of different forms of coordination in coping with work load: Cockpit versus operating theatre. Report on the psychological part of the project report on the psychological part of the project. GIHRE-Kolleg (Group interaction in high risk environments) of the Daimler-Benz-Foundation. Zurich, Switzerland: Swiss Federal Institute of Technology; 2004.

23. U.S. Medicine information central. Available at: http://www.usmedicine.com/article.cfm?articleID=896&issueID=64; 2004. Accessed June 27, 2009.

24. Haines T, Stringer B. Could the death of a BC OR nurse have been prevented by using the hands-free technique/La mort d'une infirmière de sale d'opération en Colombie-Britannique aurait-elle pu être prevenue au moyen de la technique mains libres? Can Oper Room Nurs J 2007;25(4):8, 10–11, 19–20, 22–4.

25. Stringer B, Haines T, Goldsmith CH, et al. Is use of the hands-free technique during surgery, a safe work practice, associated with safety climate? Am J Infect Control 2009;37(9):766–72.

26. Stringer B, Haines T, Oudyk J. Noisiness in operating theatres: nurses' perceptions and potential difficulty communicating. J Periop Pract 2008;18(9):384–91.

27. Folin A, Nyberg B, Nordstom G. Reducing blood exposures during orthopedic surgical procedures. AORN J 2000;71(3):573–82.

28. Stringer B, Haines T, Goldsmith CH, et al. Hands-free technique in the operating room: reduction in body fluid exposure and the value of a training video. Public Health Rep 2009;124(Suppl 1):169–79.

29. Eggleston MK, Wax JR, Philput C, et al. Use of surgical pass trays to reduce intraoperative glove perforations. J Matern Fetal Med 1997;6(4):245–7.

30. Viera AJ, Garrett JM. Understanding interobserver agreement: the kappa statistic. Fam Med 2005;37(5):360–3.

31. Stringer B, Haines T, Goldsmith CH, et al. The hands-free technique: a semi-structured interview study. AORN J 2006;84:233–48.

32. Newgard CD, Haukoos JS. Advanced statistics: missing data in clinical research—part 2: multiple imputation. Acad Emerg Med 2007;14(7):669–78.

33. Osborne S. Influences on compliance with standard precautions among operating room nurses. Am J Infect Control 2003;31(7):415–23.

34. Jeong IS, Park S. Use of hands-free technique among operating room nurses in the republic of Korea. Am J Infect Cont 2009;37(2):131–5.

35. Cunningham TR, Austin J. Using goal setting, task clarification, and feedback to increase the use of the hands-free technique by hospital operating room staff. J Appl Behav Anal 2007;40(4):673–7.
36. Centers for Disease Control and Prevention. Evaluation of blunt suture needles in preventing percutaneous injuries among health-care workers during gynecologic surgical procedures—New York City, March 1993–June 1994. MMWR Morb Mort Wkly Rep 1997;46(2):25–9. Available at: http://aepo-xdv-www.epo.cdc.gov/wonder/prevguid/m0045660/m0045660.asp. Accessed June 30, 2009.
37. Mingoli A, Sapienza P, Sgarzini G, et al. Influence of blunt needles on surgical glove perforation and safety for the surgeon. Am J Surg 1996;172(5):512–7.
38. Tanner J, Parkinson H. Double gloving to reduce surgical cross-infection [review]. Cochrane Database Syst Rev 2006;(3):CD003087.

"Scalpel Safety," not "Safety Scalpel": A New Paradigm in Staff Safety

Michael Sinnott, MBBS, FACEM, FRACP[a],*,
Ramon Shaban, BSc(Med), BN, PGDipPH&TM, GCertInfCon, DipAppSc(Amb),
MCHlth(Hons), MEd, RN, EMT-P, IPN, CICP, FRCNA[b]

KEYWORDS
• Sharps • Scalpel • Safety

SHARPS INJURIES: A PERENNIAL PROBLEM

Health care workers (HCWs) are highly susceptible to sharps injury or percutaneous injury and to acquiring a blood-borne pathogen because of their nature of work. There are as many as 1 million sharps injuries reported in the United States every year.[1] Some authorities suggest that the underreporting rate is as high as 70%,[1] meaning that the total number of injuries could be as high as 3 million per year. Many say "it won't happen to me," but HCWs know someone who will sustain a contaminated or noncontaminated sharps injury in the upcoming year.

WHAT IS THE RISK OF ACQUIRING AN INFECTION?

At least 20 pathogens have been identified as being able to be transmitted via sharps injuries in health and laboratory settings, the most common being hepatitis B and C viruses and human immunodeficiency virus (HIV).[2] Although hepatitis B and C viruses

Declaration: We declare that the contents of this article, in whole or in part, have not been previously reported and are not under consideration for publication elsewhere, nor will be, until a decision is made by *Perioperative Nursing Clinics*.

Conflict of interest: (1) Michael Sinnott is the Managing Director of QlickSmart Pty Ltd, an Australian research and development company with an emphasis on staff and patient safety, particularly with respect to sharps; (2) Ramon Shaban has no conflict of interest to declare.

Funding: No funding is associated with the preparation or publication of this article.

[a] Department of Emergency Medicine, Princess Alexandra Hospital, 199 Ipswich Road, Woolloongabba, Queensland 4102, Australia

[b] Research Centre for Clinical and Community Practice Innovation, Griffith Institute for Health and Medical Research, Griffith University and Princess Alexandra Hospital, Brisbane, Australia

* Corresponding author.

E-mail address: michael_sinnott@health.qld.gov.au

Perioperative Nursing Clinics 5 (2010) 59–67
doi:10.1016/j.cpen.2009.11.001
periopnursing.theclinics.com
1556-7931/10/$ – see front matter © 2010 Elsevier Inc. All rights reserved.

and HIV are the most feared, there is clear evidence of transmission of other significant infections. Transmission of *Plasmodium falciparum* malaria from a patient to an HCW via contaminated needlestick injury has been documented.[3] Other infections, including hepatitis D, viral hemorrhagic fever, tetanus, herpes simplex, and syphilis, have been reported.[4,5]

The seroconversion rates for an HCW who received a sharps injury from an infected patient can range from 5% to 35% for hepatitis B, 3% to 10% for hepatitis C, and 0.3% for HIV.[6] This means that when injured by a needlestick from an infected patient, the risk of seroconversion for contracting hepatitis B is as high as 1 in 3, for hepatitis C it is 1 in 10, and for HIV it is 1 in 300. However, statistics are meaningless to individual HCWs who go on to seroconvert. Although there have been significant advances in the treatment of HIV and hepatitis C, there remains no cure.

WHAT ARE THE FINANCIAL CONSEQUENCES OF SHARPS INJURIES?

The consequences for HCWs who sustain a sharps injury can be serious. The financial and human costs of occupational exposure from sharps, although difficult to quantify and qualify, are enormous. The financial impact of sharps injuries falls into 3 broad categories. First, the cost of an uncomplicated sharps injury is estimated to be as high as $3766.[7] Second, the cost of an infected sharps injury is estimated to be $100,000 annually for the treatment of HIV or hepatitis C. The cost of an injury from a scalpel cut to a digital nerve or a vessel is estimated to be $100,000, and it requires up to 3 months off work to undergo extensive rehabilitation.[8,9] The third is compensation, with the largest lawsuit to date being $12.2 million in 1998.[10]

WHAT ARE THE "HUMAN" COSTS OF SHARPS INJURIES?

The human costs of sharps injuries are myriad. The cost of loss of individual productivity and income is significant. Those who sustain sharps injuries often experience substantial and sustained psychological distress. This may range from an expected level of distress to an adjustment disorder, depression, or even posttraumatic stress disorder (PTSD). The potential psychological impact on HCWs after percutaneous injury is emphasized in an article[11] that examined 2 cases of PTSD in HCWs after needlestick exposures to HIV, even though neither seroconverted. Furthermore, there may be a negative impact on interpersonal relationships, including a need to defer plans for pregnancy. There is also an attendant risk of vertical transmission to the unborn fetus.

HOW IMPORTANT IS THIS TO PERIOPERATIVE NURSES?

Scalpel injuries account for between 7% and 12% of all sharps injuries.[12–15] There are documented cases of health care–acquired infection as a result of scalpel injury, most of which are associated with surgical dissections.[16] Historically, the focus on preventing sharps injuries has concentrated on needlestick injuries; first, because they are the most common sharps injuries, and second, because they carry higher risk of seroconversion as a consequence of the volume of blood potentially involved in the injury. However, the incidence of staff members sustaining a scalpel injury caused by those who regularly use them, such as perioperative nurses, is more than 200 times higher than their risk of suffering a needlestick injury.[17] One study reported that there were 662 sharps injuries per 100,000 scalpel blades purchased, whereas only 3.2 sharps injuries per 100,000 disposable syringes and loose needles purchased.[17]

HOW DID SAFETY LEGISLATION COME INTO EXISTENCE?

Efforts to increase the awareness of potential hazards of sharps injuries and related prevention efforts began in the early 1980s. In 1987, the US Centers for Disease Control and Prevention (CDC) issued recommendations titled "Universal Precautions" that included guidance on sharps injury prevention.[4] Universal precautions, intended to reduce exposures, relied on barriers (eg, protective gloves) and work practice controls to prevent sharps injuries. Despite these recommendations, there was only limited success in reducing the incidence of sharps injuries because of suboptimal adherence to recommendations and because most protective clothing is penetrable by sharps. Thus, additional interventions were needed to make further gains in preventing sharps injuries.[4]

A landmark 1988 study demonstrated that sharp devices that require manipulation or disassembly after use were associated with higher rates of occupational injuries.[18]

In the early 1990s, the Service Employees International Union (SEIU), which has a membership of 710,000 HCWs nationally, sent a petition to the Food and Drug Administration (FDA) requesting them to "remove from the market unsafe needles and related devices." The FDA refused to issue performance standards for needle-bearing devices and, instead, encouraged medical device manufacturers to voluntarily develop and adopt safer medical devices. On November 29, 2000, the SEIU, along with the Public Citizen, again petitioned the FDA to enforce the replacement of non-safety syringes with safety syringes.

The first sharps injury prevention law was passed in California in 1998, which was followed several years later with President Bill Clinton signing into law the Needlestick Safety and Prevention Act on November 6, 2000.[19] The first standard published in 1991 by the US Occupational Safety and Health Administration (OSHA), Regulation (Standard-29 CFR) Bloodborne pathogens-1910.1030, clarified the need for employers to select safer needle devices and to involve frontline employees in identifying and choosing these devices.[20] Recent revisions require most employers to maintain a log of injuries from contaminated sharps, enabling the institution to monitor trends, identify high-risk procedures or instruments, and measure the effectiveness of preventative efforts.[20]

LIMITATION OF ENGINEERED SHARPS INJURY PREVENTION DEVICES

The early focus on engineered sharps injury prevention (ESIP) devices seems to have delayed rather than expedited the development of optimal safety devices. ESIP required that the safety feature be built into the original device rather than be a separate purpose-built device in its own right. The potential benefits of this approach were obvious, but the unforseen downside has been very problematic; the built-in safety features have been shown to be suboptimal, and the beneficial features and function of the original device have been compromised. The CDC study, conducted from 1993 to 1995 by Alvarado-Ramy and colleagues,[21] found that 59% of injuries with ESIP devices occurred before activation of the safety feature, 20% occurred during activation, and 18% occurred when the device was not activated by the user.

Arguably a better focus on designing safety devices would be to concentrate on "passive or automatic" safety in preference to "active or manual" safety. The difference between passive safety and active safety refers to whether the safety feature is activated automatically (ie, passive safety) or it needs to be manually activated by the user (**Fig. 1**). The latter can be as simple as pressing a button or more complex, requiring a cover to be pushed over the exposed sharp after it has been used. This is best illustrated by examining safety syringes. The safest are the spring-loaded

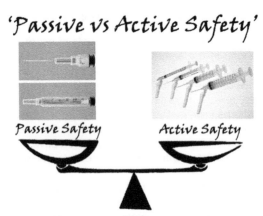

Fig. 1. Passive safety versus active safety. (*Left*) Retractable safety syringe activated automatically via a spring. (*Right*) Safety syringe activated manually, with user pushing cover over end of the needle.

retractable syringes (passive safety), in which there is automatic retraction of the sharp into the syringe after the plunger is pushed to the end of the barrel. The devices requiring a sheath to be manually pushed over the end of the needle at the completion of the procedure (active safety) are much more prone to be involved in an injury and are thus considered to be less safe. From a practical point of view, the passive safety devices are usually single handed, whereas the active safety devices usually require both hands to operate.

EXISTING PARADIGMS FOR AMELIORATING THE RISK: SAFETY SCALPELS

Most ESIP devices or safety scalpels fall into 1 of the 2 main categories: those in which the operator retracts the blade inside the handle (much like a box cutter) and those in which a sheath is moved forward or backward to cover or expose the blade. Both types are active safety devices (as apposed to passive or automatic safety devices). Despite US OSHA guidelines strongly recommending the use of ESIP devices, surgeons continue to refuse to use these active or ESIP safety scalpels citing patient safety, a lack of correct balance and feel, obstructed vision, and limited range of choice as their reasons.[22] Up to 98% of surgeons surveyed in 30 hospitals from United States and Australia disliked safety scalpels and preferred traditional handles.

The issue here is that operating room nursing staff and scrub technologists are exposed to high-risk and dangerous yet potentially preventable injuries. The other unexpected and dangerous outcome of the ESIP concept is that it leads to the widespread use of the inaccurate misnomer "safety scalpel." This name suggests that the device is safe, which is in fact far from the truth. There is no proof of safety. Early publications found that the incidence of injury with safety scalpels was higher than the incidence of injury with the traditional reusable scalpel handle. In one study between 2000 and 2001, 91 injuries were reported to be caused by reusable scalpels and 42 injuries were caused by disposable scalpels (described elsewhere in the article as safety scalpels).[10] This was incorrectly interpreted as evidence to support use of safety scalpels. However, according to Dunn, the use of safety scalpels in 2002 was only 22%.[23] This means that the incidence of injures from safety scalpels was at least twice as high as the incidence from the traditional reusable metal handle.

The Australian Safety and Efficacy Register of New Interventional Procedures published an extensive international literature review to identify and assess the efficacy of devices and procedures that are designed to lower the incidence of scalpel injuries in the operative setting.[24] They found no evidence that safety scalpels were safe. Stoker[22] found that more than three-quarters of the 57 responses reported futility in trying to make their surgeons switch to safety scalpels. One-quarter of the respondents reported blatant surgeon refusal to try safety scalpels, with 44% of surgeons reporting that they did not like them.[22] A more accurate name for these scalpels would be "retractable scalpels" or "sheathed scalpels" rather than safety scalpels.

CALLING FOR A NEW PARADIGM: "SCALPEL SAFETY," NOT "SAFETY SCALPELS"

A perfect safety system to prevent all scalpel injuries is currently beyond us. Even banning scalpels and replacing them with other implements (eg, cautery) has its own set of safety issues, such as toxic fumes. Working on the assumption that a passive safety device was the goal, whether it was completely separate from or engineered into the design of the original device, led to the development of a new wave of safety devices with better acceptance by the end user. The development of such devices involved active collaboration with primary users, namely nursing staff members, who are disproportionately represented in sharps injury statistics. Research shows convincingly that a single-handed scalpel blade remover combined with a hands-free passing technique (HFPT) is a safe alternative choice to the safety scalpel. It carries a huge practical advantage insomuch as it does not involve changing the surgeon's preference for the metal handle.

Stringer and colleagues[25] found that the use of a HFPT was effective in reducing sharps injuries from 10% to 4% in operations with greater than 100 mL of blood loss. Fuentes and colleagues[26] studied 137 scalpel injuries occurring in a 550-bed adult metropolitan tertiary referral hospital during a 16-year period from 1987 to 2003. They analyzed and compared the potential effectiveness of 2 safety strategies: safety scalpel versus a single-handed scalpel blade remover combined with a HFPT. They found that just fewer than 50% of injuries occurred while the scalpel was in use, and those injuries were assumed to be not preventable, as outlined in **Fig. 2**. Three injuries occurred when attaching the scalpel to the handle; these could have been prevented by using a safety scalpel but not by using a scalpel blade remover. However, by modeling several scenarios, using activation rates of active safety devices published by Alvarado-Ramy, Fuentes and colleagues[21] found that the combination of a single-handed scalpel blade remover and a HFPT was up to 5 times safer than a safety scalpel.

The concept of "scalpel safety" is based on providing nurses the freedom of choice to select the best safety device for their individual needs on a case-by-case basis (**Fig. 3**). Team members can now choose between a safety scalpel and a single-handed scalpel blade remover combined with a HFPT to achieve the correct balance between patient safety and staff safety.

REGULATORY UPDATE

In December 2005, OSHA published Standard Interpretations, which states that "In situations where an employer has demonstrated that the use of a scalpel with a reusable handle is required by a specific medical or dental procedure or that no alternative is feasible, the blade removal must be accomplished through the use of a mechanical device or a one-handed technique.... The use of a single-handed scalpel blade remover meets these criteria."[27] In November 2008, OSHA went on to state that

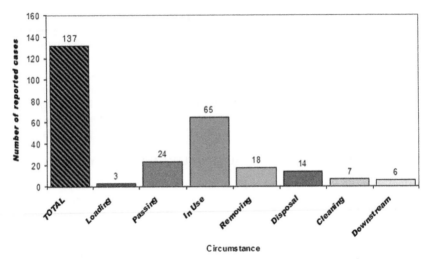

Fig. 2. Circumstances associated with scalpel blade injuries. (*Adapted from* Fuentes H, Collier J, Sinnott MJ, et al. 'Scalpel safety': modeling the effectiveness of different safety devices' ability to reduce scalpel blade injuries. Int J Risk Saf Med 2008;20:84, copyright 2008, IOS Press; with permission.)

"…using fingers to remove a used scalpel blade does not meet the requirements of the standard" and that "some facilities use a two-handed procedure with hemostat as a mechanical device to remove scalpel blades…. Hemostats have been used as a measure which was preferable to using fingers to remove a used scalpel blade. Employers are expected to consider and use safer and more effective measures when feasible."[27] With these modifications, the OSHA blood-borne pathogens guidelines in relation to scalpel blades now closely corresponds to the Australian/New Zealand Standard 3825, which is outlined in **Fig. 4.**

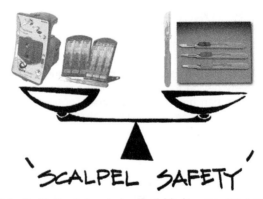

Fig. 3. Scalpel safety. (*Left*) Single-handed scalpel blade removers: nonsterile and sterile. (*Right*) Safety scalpels: sheath type and retracting type. (*Adapted from* Fuentes H, Collier J, Sinnott MJ, et al. 'Scalpel safety': modeling the effectiveness of different safety devices' ability to reduce scalpel blade injuries. Int J Risk Saf Med 2008;20:84, copyright 2008, IOS Press; with permission.)

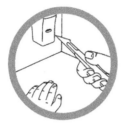

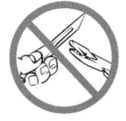

SCALPEL BLADE REMOVER
Note: This illustrates the removal of a scalpel
blade from the handle, but the design of the
illustrated scalpel blade remover does not
form part of the Standard

REMOVAL BY ARTERY FORCEPS
Note: Removal by artery forceps
or similar devices is *not* recommended

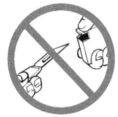

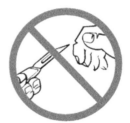

EXAMPLE OF A RESHEATHING-TYPE ACTION
Note: A resheathing-type action
is *not* recommended

REMOVAL BY HAND
Note: Removal by hand
is *not* recommended

Fig. 4. Australian standards of scalpel blade removal. (*Adapted from* Australian/New Zealand Standard 3825:1998. Procedures and devices for the removal and disposal of scalpel blades from scalpel handles, p. 6–7, copyright 1998. Reproduced with permission from SAI Global under license 0907-c036.)

An article in the March 2009 issue of the Environment of Care News by the US Joint Commission reinforces how seriously the "scalpel safety" paradigm is being taken by all American regulators, stating that traditional scalpel handles will remain the first choice of the surgeon and that to ensure staff safety, a single-handed scalpel blade remover and a HFPT will become the norm in all operating suites in the next 5 years.[28] Publication of this article suggests that the Joint Commission will be taking an active interest in the scalpel safety strategies in use when they inspect hospital operating rooms for accreditation.

SUMMARY

Nurses are too valuable to the health profession, to their patients, to their own families, and to themselves not to take their personal safety seriously. The concept of scalpel safety provides users with 2 choices: a safety scalpel or a single-handed scalpel blade remover with a HFPT. A third choice has been suggested, namely, no scalpel. However, alternative cutting devices to scalpels carry their own set of risks and costs. The correct choice should be made by the surgeon on a case-by-case basis and should consider the safety of both the patient and the staff members.

ACKNOWLEDGMENTS

Our thanks to Dr Ellen Burkett for review of this article.

REFERENCES

1. Matson K. States begin passing sharps and needle-stick legislation to protect health care workers. AORN J 2000;72(4):699–703.
2. Collins CH, Kennedy DA. Microbiological hazards of occupational needlestick and 'sharps' injuries. J Appl Bacteriol 1987;62(5):385–402.
3. Alweis R, DiRosario K, Conidi G, et al. Serial nosocomial transmission of *Plasmodium falciparum* malaria from patient to nurse to patient. Infect Control Hosp Epidemiol 2004;25(1):55–9.
4. Department of Health and Ageing. Infection control guidelines for the prevention of transmission of infectious diseases in the healthcare setting. Canberra (Australia): Commonwealth of Australia; 2004.
5. Sinnott MJ, Thomas PP, Whitby M. Herpes simplex virus: yet another risk of needlestick. Emerg Med 1997;9:339–40.
6. Doebbeling BN. Lessons regarding percutaneous injuries amongst healthcare providers. Infect Control Hosp Epidemiol 2003;24(2):82–5.
7. Lee JM, Botteman MF, Xanthakos N, et al. Needlestick injuries in the United States: epidemiologic, economic, and quality of life issues. AAOHN J 2005;53(5):117–33.
8. Davis MS. Take 'time out' for patient safety and worker safety in the OR. Adv Expo Prev 2004;7(2):22–3.
9. Jagger J, Hunt EH, Pearson RD. Estimated cost of needlestick injuries for six major needled devices. Infect Control Hosp Epidemiol 1990;11(11):584–8.
10. Perry J. Yale to pay $12.2M in largest-ever award in needlestick case. Adv Expo Prev 1998;3(3):26.
11. Worthington MG, Ross JJ, Bergeron EK. Posttraumatic stress disorder after occupational HIV exposure: two cases and a literature review. Infect Control Hosp Epidemiol 2006;27(2):215–7.
12. Argenteros PA, Castella A, Anselmo E, et al. Surgical site infection surveillance in Piedmont region, Italy. J Hosp Infect 2006;64(Suppl 1):S98–9.
13. US EPINet Needlestick and Sharps Injury Surveillance Network. Sharps Injury Data Report; 35 hospitals contributing data, 1033 total injuries. University of Virginia: International Healthcare Worker Safety Center; 2005. Available at: http://www.healthsystem.virginia.edu/internet/epinet/2005-EPINet-Needle-Stick-Data.pdf.
14. Gillen M, McNary J, Lewis J, et al. Sharps-related injuries in California healthcare facilities: pilot study results from sharps injury surveillance registry. Infect Control Hosp Epidemiol 2003;24(2):113–21.
15. Smith DR, Wei N, Zhang Y, et al. Needlestick and sharps injuries among a cross-section of physicians in mainland China. Am J Ind Med 2006;49(3):169–74.
16. Cornwall J, Singer MD. Physical injuries in the dissecting room. Clin Anat 2008; 21(1):82–5.
17. Einenstein HC, Smith DA. Epidemiology of reported sharps injuries in a tertiary care hospital. J Hosp Infect 1992;20(4):271–80.
18. Jagger J, Hunt EH, Brand-Elnaggar J, et al. Rates of needle-stick injury caused by various devices in a university hospital. N Engl J Med 1998;319:284–8.
19. Department of Health and Human Services & Centers for Disease Control and Prevention. Proceedings report. Paper presented at: National Sharps and Injury Prevention Meeting; September 12, 2005; Crown Plaza Atlanta Airport Hotel, Atlanta GA, USA.
20. Occupational Safety and Health Administration. Safety and health topics: bloodborne pathogens and needlestick prevention. Available at: http://www.osha.gov/SLTC/bloodbornepathogens/. Accessed August 21, 2009.

21. Alvarado-Ramy F, Beltrami EM, Short LJ, et al. A comprehensive approach to percutaneous injury prevention during phlebotomy: results of a multicentre study, 1993–1995. Infect Control Hosp Epidemiol 2003;24(2):97–104.

22. Stoker R. Making your scalpels safer. Outpatient Surgery 2008;IX(5):70.

23. Sinnott MJ, Wall D. Scalpel safety: how safe (or dangerous) are safety scalpels? Int J Surg 2007;6(2):176–7.

24. Royal Australasian College of Surgeons. Scalpel safety in the operative setting. Melbourne (Australia): Royal Australasian College of Surgeons; 2007. ASER-NIP-S Report 59.

25. Stringer B, Infante-Rivard C, Hanley JA. Effectiveness of the hands-free technique in reducing operating theatre injuries. Occup Environ Med 2002;59(10): 703–7.

26. Fuentes H, Collier J, Sinnott MJ, et al. 'Scalpel safety': modeling the effectiveness of different safety devices' ability to reduce scalpel blade injuries. Int J Risk Saf Med 2008;20:83–9.

27. Occupational Safety and Health Administration, United States Department of Labor. Standards Interpretations 12/22/2005 - Use of passing trays and single-handed scalpel blade remover in a surgical setting. Standard Number: 1910.1030; 1910.1030(c)(1)(iv); 1910.1030(d)(2). 2005. Available at: http://www.osha.gov/pls/oshaweb/owadisp.show_document?p_table=INTERPRETATIONS&p_id=25339. Accessed November 30, 2009.

28. Joint Commission on Accreditation of Healthcare Organizations (JCAHO). Scalpel safety—staying safe while working on the cutting edge. Environ Care News 2009;12(3):6–7.

Instrumentation for Robotic Surgery

Mary Grace Hensell, RN, BSN, CNOR[a,b,*]

KEYWORDS

- Robotic surgery • Robotic surgery instruments
- Robotic surgery instrumentation • Robotic surgical system
- Surgical technology

Technology is revolutionizing surgery in ways that were unimaginable a generation ago. Surgical technology literally resembles a science fiction movie with robots and three-dimensional (3D) devices. Minimally invasive surgery (MIS), in use for at least 20 years, is one of the precursors to robotics. Minimally invasive surgery can be described as the use of scopes and smaller incisions that use long instruments to maneuver through small areas, thus eliminating the need for large incisions.[1] With the growth of MIS came the advancement of computerized-assisted surgery (also known as image-guided surgery), surgical navigations, 3-D imaging, real timing, and sensing in the execution of surgical procedures. Then robotic surgery evolved, which requires the use of a robot and may or may not involve the direct role of the surgeon during the procedure.

Robotic surgery is defined as a computerized system that interacts with the surgical field by a mechanical arm or arms. Robotic surgery can be classified as supervisory-controlled, telesurgical, and shared-control. Supervisory-controlled robotic surgery is executed solely by the robot whose actions are determined by input from a computer program and surgeon. Telesurgical robotic surgery is manipulated by the surgeon from a remote area and uses sensor data from the robot; technically, the robot is performing the surgery. With shared-control systems, such as the da Vinci Surgical System (Intuitive Surgical, Inc, Sunnyvale, CA, USA [Intuitive]) the surgeon controls and performs the procedure and the robot offers different manipulations, such as a 360° articulation, and increases steadiness of hands, thereby eliminating tremors.[1]

HISTORY OF ROBOTIC SURGICAL SYSTEMS

An important early contributor to the development of robotic surgery technology was a medical device company, Computer Motion, founded in 1989. The company's first robot, Aesop, was designed to hold an endoscopic camera in minimally invasive

^a Allegheny General Hospital, 320 East North Avenue, Pittsburgh, PA 15212, USA
^b 722 Midway Drive, Pittsburgh, PA 15126, USA
* 722 Midway Drive, Pittsburgh, PA 15126.
E-mail address: mhensell722@comcast.net

Perioperative Nursing Clinics 5 (2010) 69–81
doi:10.1016/j.cpen.2009.12.002   periopnursing.theclinics.com
1556-7931/10/$ – see front matter. Published by Elsevier Inc.

laparoscopic surgery and was operated by foot pedals. The third arm eliminated tremors while holding the camera. In 1993, Aesop 1000 became the first visual aid robotic surgical device approved by the US Food and Drug Administration (FDA). In 1996, Aesop 2000 was marketed with voice instead of foot pedal control.[2]

After several more Aesop models, the Zeus Robotic Surgical System was the next improvement, with three robotic arms attached onto the side of the operating room (OR) bed. Zeus was approved by the FDA in 2001 and used a joystick to control its arms. This system featured the microjoint, designed to hold 28 different instruments, including scalpels, hooks, scissors, and dissectors. Zeus was specifically designed to complete endoscopic cardiac surgical procedures, such as coronary artery bypass grafts.[2]

Next-generation developments included Hermes, which used intelligent tools and not robotic arms, and Socrates, which used a telesurgical system. In 1995, Intuitive Surgical was formed based on technology developed by the Stanford Research Institute. Intuitive Surgical collaborated with several institutions and companies to create the daVinci Surgical System. In 1997 the daVinci Surgical System got FDA approval to assist in surgery and in July 2000 it became the first laparoscopic surgical robotic system to receive FDA clearance to perform surgery. This system's contributions to robotics are the EndoWrist and a 3-D vision system. These features provide high precision, flexibility, and the ability to articulate 360° in tiny areas.[2] This robotic system has been FDA-approved for many types of surgery, including general surgery procedures (eg, cholecystectomy, gastric bypass, Roux-en-Y, Whipple, Nissen fundoplication); urological procedures (eg, radical prostatectomy, cystectomy, nephrectomy, pyeloplasty, sacrocolpopexy); gynecologic procedures (eg, tubal ligation, ovarian cystectomy, hysterectomy, myomectomy); cardiac surgical procedures (eg, coronary artery bypass graft, valve replacements); and thoracic procedures (eg, fundoplications). Because robots do not replace human beings but rather improve their ability to operate through smaller incisions, they allow surgeons to access areas of the body that their hands could not previously maneuver into.

ADVANTAGES AND DISADVANTAGES

Some advantages of the robot are that it reduces hospital stays by approximately half, reducing cost approximately 33%. Still other advantages include significant decrease in blood loss, decreased pain, smaller incisions, decreased scarring, and quicker recovery.[3] Of particular note is the nerve-sparing advantage of robotic prostatectomy, which decreases the postoperative complication of impotence.[4] Use of the robotic arm has advantages and disadvantages for surgeons, as indicated in **Table 1**.

Because robotic surgeries are so integrated with computers and advanced imaging techniques, their proper use requires an immense amount of training resulting in a steep learning curve.[5,6] Many surgeons initially feel hindered by the loss of tactile sensation (ability to feel the tissue while they operate). Robotic surgery takes approximately 45 minutes longer than comparable open procedures, but this is largely attributed to the learning curve, and surgical times are expected to improve with more experience with these systems.[3]

Any technological malfunction creates the potential for injuries. Manufacturers have attempted to reduce these risks through redundant sensors and safety features. For example, if the surgeon removes his or her head from the console viewer, the robot locks up and cannot be activated unless a head is engaged in the console viewer. During the procedure, a zero-point movement system prevents the robot's arms from pivoting at above the incision line, so that the skin cannot be torn.[3] Included in

Table 1
Advantages and disadvantages of using the robotic arm for surgeons

Advantages	Disadvantages
Articulates 360 degrees	Currently limited to simple procedures
Reduces hand tremors and fatigue	Expensive
Scales large movements to smaller ones	Limited eye-hand coordination
3-D imaging	Difficult to construct and debug Potential computer faulting
Decreased potential for infection	Advanced training Large learning curve
Precise movements	Increased surgical time in the beginning

the power source is a battery backup that allows the system to run for 20 minutes. The machine needs to be plugged in at all times and on a dedicated circuit; it requires a 24-hour charge to be functional again. There is an emergency stop button that stops all movement of the robot in case of emergencies. The robot can be disengaged manually if it faults, and there is an override button so that surgery can be continued. Although highly desirable, all of these safety features contribute to the cost of the robot, which is prohibitively high for some institutions.[3]

COMPONENTS

The most commonly used robotic surgical system, the da Vinci, has several models: the first generation model, the S system, and the newest model, the HD. The drapes and equipment for each of the models have small variations and are not interchangeable. The da Vinci Surgical System has four major components: the surgeon console, robot, detachable instruments, and 3-D vision system.[3,5,6] When setting up the system, the cables need to be connected appropriately; these connections are color coded to prevent connecting the vision system, console, and robot incorrectly. When completing different surgeries in different surgical services, positioning of the equipment becomes extremely important because the equipment cannot be easily moved.

The vision system (**Fig. 1**) has a high resolution because of the 3-D endoscope, and is equipped with two independent vision channels on its endoscope, linking the image back to the monitor. This feature provides the true-to-life 3-D images of the operative field. The video system also incorporates a high-performance video camera and audio equipment on the tower with voice controls. Operating images are enhanced, refined, and optimized using image synchronizers, high-intensity illuminators, and camera control units.[3] This enhancement results in a high-resolution 3-D image that is bright, crisp, and clear, with no fatigue-inducing flicker or cross fading as is common with single-monitor systems.

The vision cart holds two white-balance components; the white balance should be in the 12-o'clock position; the first generation robot system has a black balance and there is also a focusing component. Additionally, there is an illuminator, and an extra bulb should be available because of the limited amount of hours available on the bulb (500 hours). The illuminator has a higher intensity then regular light sources. The light source should be placed on standby when not in use but not turned off because it takes 30 minutes to reboot. There is an audio control that attaches to the console so that the physician's voice can be delivered to the room from the vision cart. The monitors have a touch-screen scope alignment (**Fig. 2**) and a surgistrate. This feature

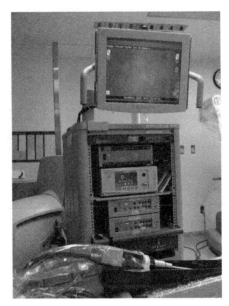

Fig. 1. Vision system cart.

permits the surgeon to outline (with a finger on the monitor screen) the area to dissect or cut; the outline appears on the console screen. This process, similar to marking football maneuvers on a chalkboard, can be used to teach other surgeons where dissection should take place.[5,6]

The next piece of equipment is the surgeon console (**Fig. 3**). The surgeon operates while seated at the console, positioned several feet from the OR bed, allowing him or her to have a magnified 3-D image of the surgical field. The surgeon's head tilts into the viewer and the surgeon's hands grasp the controls on the system's master interface.[3] This interface seamlessly translates the surgeon's wrist and finger movements into precise real-time movements of the surgeon. There are foot pedals that have focusing pedals and clutches to switch to the different arms, because not all the arms can be used at the same time.[5,6]

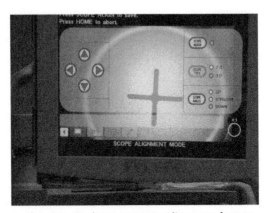

Fig. 2. Monitor screen showing touch-screen scope alignment feature.

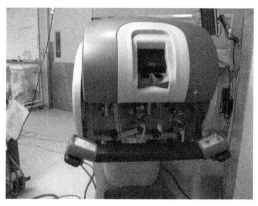

Fig. 3. Surgeon's console. Note the control pods on the left and right side of the armrest.

The console has a power button on the right pod (**Fig. 4**); once powered up the system will go through a 30-second electrical test. The surgeon should not place her or his head into the viewer during the test. After the arms of the robot are extended, the machine is homed from the console. The robot will go through a series of arm movements and it will emit three chirps that indicate that it is homed. The left pod (**Fig. 5**) has additional controls where the surgeon can manually align the scope, override a fault, adjust scaling, and silence the alarm. The height of the head can be adjusted on the side of the console.[5,6]

The robot (**Fig. 6**) has two or three instrument arms and one endoscope arm. A fourth instrument arm is available, allowing manipulation of another instrument for complex procedures.[3] All available arms are not used in all surgeries; surgical team members can swing unused arms to the right or left side by releasing a locking mechanism located on the main post of the robot. The robot is motorized but has a drive and a neutral toggle on the base. The robot can be moved manually by the middle pivot on the base, which controls the direction of the robot. The pivot should be swung in the opposite direction of that which the robot is to be moved. The arms can be clutched and moved by pressing the button on the top side of the arm, which moves the arm

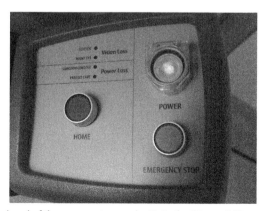

Fig. 4. Right control pod of the surgeon's console. Note the "Home," "Power," and "Emergency Stop" buttons.

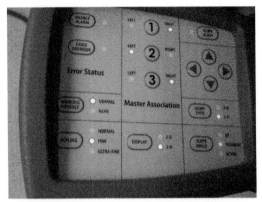

Fig. 5. Left control pod of the surgeon's console, with various control features, such as fault status and type of scope angle.

outwards; the button also has an LED light that, when illuminated in blue, indicates the instrument can be pushed downward along the shaft into the abdomen. On the main part of the arm is another clutch that moves the arm side to side.[5,6]

The detachable instruments allow the robot arms to simulate fine human movements. Each instrument has a particular function; instruments can be changed from one to another, using quick-release levers on each robot arm. The position of the robotic arm is memorized before an instrument is removed so that the replacement can be reset to the same position. The instruments can rotate in full circles and have seven degrees of freedom (ie, the number of independent movements the robot can perform). The surgeon is also able to control the amount of force applied, and the robotic technology can filter out hand tremors and scale the surgeon's large hand movements into smaller ones.[3]

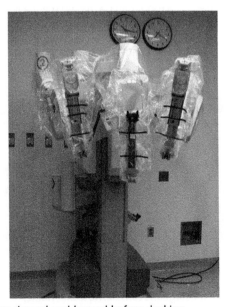

Fig. 6. Robot with arms draped and homed before docking.

MAINTENANCE

The console viewer, armrest, and master controllers can be cleaned with antibacterial soap, water, and a nonabrasive cloth. The outside of the components can be cleaned with a disinfectant. The connections should be kept covered by a metal cover made by the manufacturer. The connection cable should be periodically cleaned inside with a manufacturer-recommended cleaner, using several drops of the cleaner placed onto a pipe cleaner and dusted inside along the connection points. The bulb on the illuminator should be checked for number of hours of use. All other recommended maintenance activities necessary to maintain the warranties should be performed. The robot can also be wiped with an approved hospital disinfectant.[5,6]

HANDLING SYSTEM COMPONENTS

It is highly recommended to house the robot in one OR room; moving it is difficult because it is very heavy and cumbersome. Care should be taken if moving the components, such as pulling the vision cart appropriately and making sure that someone assists with doors, because the electrical components could easily be damaged by minor impacts. When moving the console, the wrist rest should not be pulled because it contains electrical sensors that may be damaged. Likewise, the robot's arms should be moved only when clutched; the robot arms must be confined when moving the robot so that they are not bumped. The robot itself is motorized but can also be placed into neutral and moved manually. It is recommended not to toggle frequently from neutral to drive on the base of the robot because these toggles break easily, necessitating a 1- to 2-day repair because the robot has to be lifted up to fix the gears that are located under the base.[5,6]

DRAPING CONSIDERATIONS: DRAPES AS INSTRUMENT COMPONENTS

Draping the robot is very similar to draping a microscope except that the drape for the robot has a sterile adapter. What is unique about the drapes for the robot arms is that the adapter can be considered part of the instrument and the drapes can be billed for as an instrument cost.

To drape the robot, lower a drape over one arm of the robot, place the sterile adapter, and slide it down into the arm carriage. Using both thumbs, push the sterile adapter into the instrument arm until it clicks. The wheels on the sterile adapter will spin and three beeps signal that the system recognizes the adapter. Continue to drape the arm like a microscope. Bend the drape's flexible strips to create a clear path for the instrument to slide down against (**Fig. 7**). Remember when draping the robot to start at the farthest end and work toward you to avoid contaminating yourself or the other drapes. Continue draping the arms until you get to the camera head.[5,6]

Locate the sweet spot (a designated area on the upper arm) before draping the camera head. The sweet spot maintains alignment of the robot arms. Lower the camera drape over the arm and install the sterile camera mount by aligning the pins to the reinforced section of the drape. Keep the paper above the camera mount because the camera gets very hot and can melt the drape if the paper reinforcement is removed. Bend the flexible strips to create a clear path for the camera and continue draping up the arm.[5,6]

The endoscope is draped next. The sterile adapter is attached to the endoscope and taped onto the tan adapter, and the scope end sticks out of the drape. The circulator holds the camera and the scrub person guides the scope onto the camera and screws it down. The scrub person connects the double-ended light cord to the scope

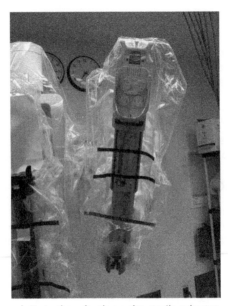

Fig. 7. Robot arm, draped. Note the wheels on the sterile adapter.

and the drape is maneuvered down the lengthy cords toward the circulator. The most common mistake is to drape backward; the drape is to cover the cords, not the scope, so it appears to be backward. A separate table is needed for the camera, light cord, and scope. The author recommends a Cysto cart because it has sides that will not permit the serpentine light cord to fall off the table (**Fig. 8**). Additionally, the light cord and camera are awkward and heavy; they are less likely to be damaged if they are placed on a separate table.[5,6]

ROBOTIC SURGERY INSTRUMENTATION

Robotic surgery instrumentation is similar to laparoscopic instruments; in fact the tips of the instruments are the same as other laparoscopic instrumentation. The base

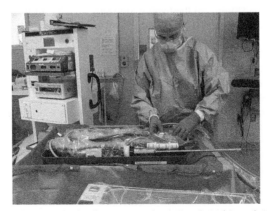

Fig. 8. Scrub person draping the endoscope cord. Notice that this task is being performed on a draped table with sides to contain the coiled cord.

(housing unit) of the instrument contains microchips. A daVinci EndoWrist instrument comprises the housing unit and the shaft; the instrument name is printed on the front of the housing unit or base (eg, large needle driver, 8 mm). On either side of the housing unit are release levers to connect and disconnect from the drape and the robot. The instrument shaft is covered in a black silicone-type material to protect the electronics within the shaft, and is similar in length to other laparoscopic instruments. Proximal to the tip of the instrument is the wrist, which can articulate or move the instrument tip. The tip delineates the type of instrument, such as needle drive or scissor (**Fig. 9**).[5,6]

On the housing unit are two flush ports. On the back of the housing unit are four pulley-type wheels that attach to the instrument drape and robot (**Fig. 10**). Similar to other laparoscopic cases, a 0° endoscope is required, but robotic surgery necessitates a 30° scope camera that has 3-D capability, unlike the usual capabilities of a two-dimensional camera and scope. A camera adapter is supplied to connect the scope and camera to each other, and a bifurcated light cord connects the scope to the high-intensity light source. One can see the similarities to other traditional laparoscopic instrumentation but there are key differences with the scope, cameras, and light sources as described earlier. The scope can be immersed only in water, never saline, and a scope warmer is recommended (**Fig. 11**).[5,6]

Because of the learning curve and extended surgical time, a toggle switch on the insufflator is recommended because the need to switch to a second tank of compressed gas is common; this prevents loss of pneumoperitoneum. As with all surgery, the scrub person should inspect the instrumentation for instrument damage, and the circulator should inspect all the connections on the machines. During the case, the scrub person should flush the second port to keep the instrument clean and free from clogging. The instruments should be wiped with sterile water and kept free from debris, similar to other cases.[5,6]

The instruments are maneuvered by an intricate pulley system within the robot's arms, so it is imperative that the pulley wheels are free to move without limitations. The scrub person should press the pulleys to see that the pulleys are free from constraints. This step should also be completed when draping the robot to keep the pulleys loose and able to function.[5,6]

Some robotic instruments are considered reposable and are good for 10 uses. It is recommended to keep track of the uses so that instruments can be ordered in an appropriate timeframe (5–10 days). Currently, marking with a permanent marker on

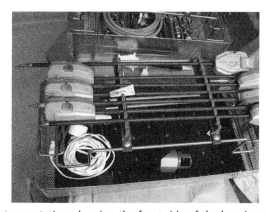

Fig. 9. Robotic instrumentation, showing the front side of the housing units.

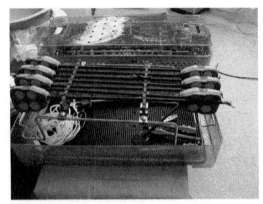

Fig. 10. Robotic instruments, showing the back side of the housing units.

the housing unit is recommended; additionally, the computer keeps track of the instrument uses. The countdown is registered and can be visualized on the vision cart monitor. The problem with relying on the computer for tracking this count is that usually a hospital will have at least two sets of robotic surgery instruments and one or two extras in case of contamination of an instrument. Every time an instrument is engaged onto the robot, it counts as another use, even if it is the first use for this instrument. Therefore, a manual count may be more accurate.[5,6]

A unique feature of the daVinci Surgical System is that not all other instrumentation can be used with the robot. The manufacturer has contractual agreements with other companies whose instrumentation was made compatible with the daVinci, including Gyrus, which carries the PK dissector and the harmonic scalpel also used for dissection.

Basic instrumentation for urologic, general, and gynecologic surgery is as follows

- daVinci Maryland
- Large needle holder X2
- Mega needle holder, prograsper
- PK dissector (Gyrus)
- Scissors

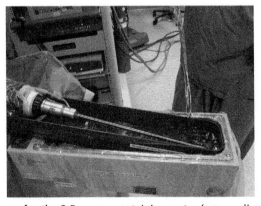

Fig. 11. Scope warmer for the 3-D scope, containing water (never saline).

- Cadieree forceps
- Hot shears
- Hook cautery
- Double fenestrated grasper (particular to general surgery)
- Scissor cover.

Additionally, a precise bipolar cautery may be ordered if the PK dissectors from Gyrus are being used; this is particular to hysterectomies. A tenaculum forcep and suture cut scissors may also be ordered for gynecologic surgery.

A cobra grasper is not a necessity but instrumental to making the case go more smoothly, particularly in urology. A bowel grasper is essential for general and gyneco-logic cases. Still other instruments may be acquired depending on the specific case, such as a bladeless obturator for the trocars, daVinci trocars and seals, hot shears cover, Verstep ports, Veres needle, and Ectolube, which reduces the amount of eschar. The tools to align the endoscope are necessities for general, urologic, and gynecologic surgery.

Regular instrument sets should be assembled for urologic, gynecologic, and general surgery cases, such as a laparotomy tray with hemostats, Kellys, Allises, Kochers, scissors, needle holders, Debakeys, Adsons, Army-Navys, Richardsons, S retractors, knife handles, rulers, suctions tips, a smoke evacuator, and a stopcock. A traditional laparoscopy set should also be available in case the surgeon aborts the robotic proce-dure and needs to complete a traditional laparoscopy or laparotomy.[5,6]

If a robotic procedure must quickly be converted to an open procedure, the robot's arms are released from the trocars and then the robot can be undocked or backed out of position. Docking or undocking the robot is similar to driving a semitrailer. The robot for prostatectomies and hysterectomies is docked between patients' legs while in lithotomy position. The author recommends purchasing at least two wrenches and sterilizing them in case the robot's arms cannot be released. A sterile wrench can be placed onto the sterile field where the scrub and physician can unlock the trocars so that that the robot can be removed quickly if conversion to an open procedure is necessary.[5,6]

Cardiac instrumentation from Intuitive should include a Potts scissor, small clip applier, diamond micro forceps, round tooth forceps, Debakey forceps, Cichon tissue forceps, fine tip forceps, snap fit instrument, EndoPass delivery instrument, microbi-polar forceps, curved scissors, Resano forceps, internal mammary artery stabilizer, pericardial dissector, atrial retractor, valve hook, and cautery spatula instrument in addition to Intuitive instruments from the other services, with the exception of the bowel grasper. Regular cardiac instrument trays should be added to the sets in case the surgeon would need to convert to a sternal incision. A sternal saw should also be in the room. In cardiac surgery, patients are in a lateral position and three ports are used: one camera port at the fifth intercostal space, the right instrument arm placed at the third intercostal space, and lastly the left instrument placed at the seventh intercostal space.[5,6]

SYSTEM SHUT-DOWN PROCEDURE

At the end of all procedures is a system shut down and it has to occur in a certain sequence, similar to the start-up sequence. The author recommends marking the vision cart "first on and last off." Fold all arms of the robot to condense the storing area and store the fourth arm in the back. It folds up similar to a serpentine. Press the power button on the right-sided pod; the system will have a 10-second shut-down process and a message will appear on the vision cart stating "shut down." Power off the vision cart and disconnect the cables.[5,6]

INSTRUMENT CLEANING AND DISINFECTION

Cleaning the daVinci instruments is important to maintain proper instrument function, particularly in the housing of the instrument. A special cleaning guide is provided to the surgical facility from Intuitive that has specific instructions on how to clean the instruments. A Luer fitting attaches to the water line; which the company suggests for connecting to the flush ports. Flush the main port for at least 20 seconds, using pressurized water at a minimum of 30 psi. While flushing the instrument, hold the tip down and move the instrument wrist around in its full range of motion. Continue flushing until the water exiting is clear. Flush the remaining ports the same way until clear. Rinse the ports with an enzymatic cleaner and place the instrument into an ultrasonic bath containing an enzymatic cleaner for 15 to 45 minutes. Then repeat the flush again. Rinse the outside of the instrument thoroughly to remove the residual debris or cleaning agents. Start at the tip and then pay particular attention to the housing unit. After cleaning, dry the outside of the instrument with a lint-free cloth. Dry the inside of the instrument by injecting 71% isopropyl alcohol through the ports, then blow pressurized air through the ports. Lubricate the tip and wrist mechanism with a neutral-pH, steam-permeable lubricant, and then sterilize.[5,6]

Sterilization recommendations are for pre-vacuum steam autoclaving at 270 to 272°F or 132 to 134°C. The minimum exposure time is 4 minutes with an average dry time of 20 minutes; allow the instruments to dry following steam sterilization. The use of flash sterilization is not recommended. Do not sterilize over 285°F or 140°C. Ethylene oxide, hydrogen peroxide, and chlorine are caustic to robotic instruments, and processes that use these agents should not be used.[5,6]

ECONOMIC ISSUES

Some pertinent billing obstacles are the fact that Intuitive instrumentation is reposable and has 10 uses. The average cost of each instrument is between $2200 and $2400. To recoup some of this cost, the cost of the drapes needs to be billed in addition to the instrumentation. The drape includes the instrument adapter, so it is billable, as previously discussed. Hospitals bill in different ways. Some facilities itemize, others bill in tiers, and still others bill in 15-minute increments. However your facility bills, the most important thing is to bill for the instrumentation and divide it by 10 uses per instrument. For example, if three instruments were used for a prostatectomy at $2200 apiece, the bill should reflect $660. Additionally, in whatever method the facility uses to bill for drapes, modules, and case carts, the key consideration is that the drapes need to be built into the cost to offset the expenses for robotic procedures.

SUMMARY

Robotic surgery is here to stay and will continue to grow in use as more surgeons and teams are trained in robotics. It will not be long before more complex surgeries and possible telesurgery will occur, which will allow surgeons to operate with precise electronic connections when separated from patients by long distances. Maybe some day we will operate on astronauts in outer space. The surgical robot is a precise mechanism that requires special instrumentation, training, and care. Teams will continue to be educated to provide the best care possible to patients. The stress, blood loss, and insults upon the body from surgery will be reduced because of robotic surgery. Hospitals stays will be reduced and refinements of surgery will continue. The robotic system is redefining minimally invasive surgery by, in the words of Intuitive Surgical, "taking surgical precision and technique beyond the limits of the human hand."[7]

REFERENCES

1. Brown University. Robotic surgery: overview. Available at: http://biomed.brown.edu/Courses/BI108/BI108_2005_Groups/04/index.html. Accessed October 30, 2009.
2. Brown University. Robotic surgery: important historic robotic companies and systems. Available at: http://biomed.brown.edu/Courses/BI108/BI108_2005_Groups/04/history.html. Accessed October 30, 2009.
3. Brown University. Robotic surgery: da Vinci Surgical System. Available at: http://biomed.brown.edu/Courses/BI108/BI108_2005_Groups/04/davinci.html. Accessed October 30, 2009.
4. Brown University. Robotic surgery: urology. Available at: http://biomed.brown.edu/Courses/BI108/BI108_2005_Groups/04/urology.html. Accessed October 30, 2009.
5. Jayjohn L. Robotic specialist training program [course manual]. Sunnyvale (CA): Intuitive Surgical, Inc; 2008.
6. Jayjohn L. daVinci allied health and nurse training program [course manual]. Columbus (OH): The Ohio State University; 2008.
7. Intuitive Surgical, Inc. Endowrist instruments. Available at: http://www.intuitivesurgical.com/products/endowrist_instruments/index.aspx. Accessed October 30, 2009.

Teaching Surgical Instrumentation: Innovative Techniques

Amy L. Kennedy, RN, MSN, CNOR[a],*,
Kathleen B. Gaberson, PhD, RN, CNOR, CNE, ANEF[b]

KEYWORDS

- Surgical instruments • Teaching instrumentation
- Instruction design • Learning domains

Introducing surgical instruments to the novice perioperative nurse, nursing student, or surgical technology student is usually an interesting challenge. The novice in either discipline is usually overwhelmed by the immense array of instruments. The novice's first day in the operating room will have him or her wondering how the team makes the procedure progress so smoothly and how the scrub person and circulator know exactly what the surgeon needs at the sterile field.

To use instruments appropriately, learners need to have a basic understanding of how instruments are designed and manufactured, how they are organized for use, and the function of each instrument. Knowledge of human anatomy and tissue types is also essential. A review of learning domains and selected learning and teaching principles provides guidance for selecting appropriate learning activities to teach surgical instrumentation and designing evaluation strategies to assess that learning.

DOMAINS OF LEARNING

When designing instruction for learners, teachers must keep in mind that learning occurs in three domains: cognitive, psychomotor, and affective. Although learning for successful transfer to an actual clinical setting represents an integration of these domains, it is useful to consider them separately for planning instruction and evaluation strategies. Within each domain, learning objectives should be carefully chosen to match the level at which learners will be expected to demonstrate the abilities. Each domain has one or more taxonomies (classification systems) that organize expected outcomes from lower to higher levels of abilty.[1]

---

[a] Program of Surgical Technology, Harrisburg Area Community College, One HACC Drive, Harrisburg, PA 17110, USA
[b] OWK Consulting, 213 Sharon Drive, Pittsburgh, PA 15221, USA
* Corresponding author.
E-mail address: alkenned@hacc.edu

Perioperative Nursing Clinics 5 (2010) 83–88
doi:10.1016/j.cpen.2009.12.001
1556-7931/10/$ – see front matter © 2010 Elsevier Inc. All rights reserved.

COGNITIVE DOMAIN

Cognitive abilities relate to knowledge and intellectual skills. The most widely used taxonomy for the cognitive domain was developed by Bloom and colleagues.[2] It classifies six levels of cognitive learning with increasing complexity:

- Knowledge
- Comprehension
- Application
- Analysis
- Synthesis
- Evaluation.

Applying this taxonomy to learning surgical instruments, it is evident that learners need not only to recognize or recall the name of the instrument (knowledge) but also to understand its function (comprehension). Understanding instrument function prepares learners to be more effective and efficient in the scrub and circulating roles, and helps them anticipate the needs of the personnel working at the sterile field. Relating why a surgeon requests a particular instrument to the type of tissue being handled is an example of the analysis level of the cognitive domain. Learning objectives and related learning activities at the application level help learners develop critical thinking skills in the scrub role. For instance, anticipating the need to change from a 7-in forceps to a 9-in forceps is based on analysis of the location of the procedure, the size of the patient, and the progress of the procedure.

AFFECTIVE DOMAIN

The affective domain involves the development of values, beliefs, and attitudes. The taxonomy for this domain is based on the principle that learners progress from the awareness of a values to consistent behavior based on internalization of that value. To internalize a value and use it as the basis for decisions and actions, learners must first know what values and attitudes are important for their practice—a cognitive base. Next, learners must accept these beliefs, attitudes, and values; be motivated to use them consistently; and then use them in practice.[1]

The most widely used taxonomy for the affective domain was developed by Krathwohl and colleagues.[3] This taxonomy includes five levels of learning:

- Receiving
- Responding
- Valuing
- Organization
- Characterization by a value.

Learning goals and activities in this domain related to surgical instrumentation would begin with awareness of important values in perioperative practice (receiving). For example, the learner must understand that the patient is the center of focus for the entire surgical team and that patient safety depends on consistent use of the surgical conscience by all team members. This involves being sensitive to the needs and rights of others. Next, the learner reacts to a situation (responding), reflecting a voluntary choice. In the educational setting, learners might express their reactions to observing actions of surgical team members that are congruent and incongruent with this value. The next level is to accept and internalize a value and make a commitment to use it in practice (valuing). Learners demonstrate this level of the affective domain by consistently acting based on the internalized value. For example, learners might express concern about patient safety to their instructors or supervisors if instruments are routinely being flash sterilized as a means of compensating for low inventory. The highest levels of the affective taxonomy, organization and characterization by a value, typically are not achieved by novices in the perioperative setting because they develop over time with practice.

PSYCHOMOTOR DOMAIN

The psychomotor domain relates to developing motor skills and competency in using technology. It is important to recognize that psychomotor skills have a cognitive base because learners must understand the principles that underlie each skill. Psychomotor skills also have an affective component that reflects the values of the person who performs the skill.[1] One taxonomy for the psychomotor domain was developed by Dave.[4] Categories progress from lower to higher levels of skill:

- Imitation
- Manipulation
- Precision
- Articulation
- Naturalization.

In this domain, learners first learn by following the teacher's example of how instruments should be handled (imitation)—but this level of learning is insufficient for actual clinical practice in the role of perioperative nurse or surgical technologist. Learners must practice assembling and handling instruments following procedures (manipulation) and, after receiving feedback on their skill level, perform more accurately (precision) and within a reasonable timeframe (articulation). Developing a high level of proficiency (naturalization) in identifying, handling, passing, and caring for instruments occurs over time with repeated practice in the role.

EFFECTIVE APPROACHES TO TEACHING SURGICAL INSTRUMENTATION

In my classes, I begin to introduce a few instruments the very first day. I bring in an entire tray and pull instruments out while demonstrating and identifying what is being passed around the classroom. Many of us are visual and kinesthetic learners. We learn by seeing and learn even better by touching and handling. Introducing a few basic instruments very early in the educational program or orientation helps learners to recognize them easily when they are in the operating room observing or assisting with counts. For example, passing a hemostat and a Debakey forceps around the classroom while identifying each instrument and talking about the classification, what each is used for, what trays it will be found in, and how to pass it to the surgeon, captures learners' attention. Opening a ratchet with one hand (especially the nondominant hand) for the first time is frustrating for learners. An early demonstration and opportunity to practice and return the demonstration helps them to feel more confident in their abilities during their first experiences as members of the perioperative team. Small successes like this reinforce learning and stimulate learners' interest in learning more.

There are many great resources available to assist students in learning to recognize instruments and to assist educators in facilitating the process. Many photographic textbooks depict instruments individually or in sets, and provide the common name and aliases. Some texts include a CD or DVD that provides opportunities for independent, self-directed learning activities, individually or in pairs or groups. For example, at their own pace and at a time convenient to them, learners may use flash cards to identify names of instruments and determine what procedure the instruments would be used for, or practice setting up a Mayo stand. Some DVDs identify instruments, categories, and care and handling (decontamination and sterilization), and review the manufacturing process.

Perioperative textbooks all include information on instrumentation. Each varies slightly. Some provide a brief historical perspective; others include information on the manufacturing process and the care and handling of instruments. Textbooks may address basic and specialty instruments in this section. Others address instrumentation specific to the surgical area being addressed. Most textbooks review instrument form and function. The Program of Surgical Technology at Harrisburg Area Community College, we require students to purchase two perioperative textbooks and one instrument text. We also have available other instrument textbooks that students may borrow. Often they find other textbooks that they like and order them on their own. Our main goal in the first semester is to introduce the student to basic general surgery instruments. We then add the specialty instruments as we study those procedures. We have changed instrument textbooks several times because they keep improving and adding more interactive features. Today's students expect great photographs and other resources to assist their initial learning process and to use as clinical references throughout their education. See the representative list of available textbooks, not meant to be exhaustive, in **Box 1**.

Making instruments and sets available for learners to create their own flash cards with their digital cameras is another option. This is done in the educational setting or in the sterilization department. Some sterilization departments have their count sheets saved as computer files with photographs of the instrument trays or individual instruments with instructions for assembly. Encouraging learners to use these resources independently and providing time for them to form study groups to quiz each other on instrumentation enhances their learning and increase their self-confidence.

Providing print copies of basic and specialty instrument tray count sheets is another method of assisting learners. Usually, COUNT sheets are easily obtained from the clinical site. They help learners understand why accurate instrument counts are important for the delivery of perioperative care. Trays are commonly assembled using count

---

Box 1
Representative list of textbooks with surgical instrumentation content

Nemitz R. Surgical instrumentation: an interactive approach. St. Louis, MO: Saunders; 2010.

Rutherford C. Differentiating surgical instruments. Philadelphia, PA: F.A. Davis; 2005.

Wells M. Surgical instruments: a pocket guide. 3rd edition. St Louis, MO: Saunders; 2006.

Fuller J. Surgical technology: principles and practices. 4th edition. St. Louis, MO: Elsevier Saunders; 2005.

Rothrock J. Alexander's care of the patient in surgery. 13th edition. St. Louis, MO: Mosby Elsevier; 2007.

Fortunato N. Berry & Kohn's operating room technique. 11th edition. St Louis, MO: Mosby; 2007.

Tighe S. Instrumentation for the operating room. 7th edition. St. Louis, MO: Mosby; 2007.

Frey K. Surgical technology for the surgical technologist. 3rd edition. New York, NY: Delmar; 2008.

sheets, so students find that they are helpful from an organizational standpoint in the clinical setting and a great study tool.

Out-of-date, discarded instrument catalogs are found in most operating rooms, surgical material management departments, or sterilization departments. Learners may cut them apart and use the photographs to create their own, inexpensive sets of flash cards.

Teaching learners about the history of surgery and instruments and basic information about how instruments are manufactured promotes a greater appreciation of the importance of the care and handling of surgical instruments and the great expense of repairing instruments. Acquainting learners with the cost of just a few instruments provides them with the rationale for why the need for careful care and handling of surgical instruments is emphasized. Instruments must be in proper working order during the surgical procedure to ensure patient safety.

The sterile processing unit or department is a great learning lab for novice perioperative nurses and surgical technology students. It provides learners with an understanding of what goes on behind the scenes in the decontamination and sterilization area. Time in this area provides the learner with hands-on experience with instruments and assembling trays. This experience further reinforces the learner's knowledge and understanding of the importance of instrumentation and reinforces what has been taught regarding the decontamination and sterilization process.

In the program's surgical technology lab, we have the advantage of being able to display a basic tray of instruments with index cards labeling each instrument. This is available for the students the first few days of class. This area is available to students to study, take photographs, and handle the instruments. The students are informed when the instrument identification test will take place. This paper-and-pencil test requires that students identify the instruments and their functions. Correct spelling of instrument names is part of the test score. We also evaluate knowledge of instrumentation in a simulation environment. When students are completing competencies in a mock surgery setting, the "surgeon" (instructor) requests an instrument. To earn a satisfactory grade, students must pass the correct instrument in the correct manner. Scores in both of these areas are part of students' lab scores for the semester.

Throughout the time of preparing students to scrub for their first case in the operating room, we review local names (aliases) of instruments. Local names change from facility to facility, and from region to region. We also acquaint students with the common hand signals. These are commonly missed by the new "scrub" who tends to be preoccupied with the back table. We encourage learners new to the scrub role to direct their attention to the operative field. The clinical preceptor evaluates the student's progress. Instrument identification is an integral part of that evaluation on a daily and weekly basis. Students, as a rule, are quick to come back to class or lab and report if there are instruments that they are unfamiliar with or are struggling with passing to the surgeon or assistant. We then review the skills in the lab setting.

During lab time, we teach students the hands-free passing technique for sharps and strongly encourage them to practice using this technique. We do teach students how to pass sharps, knowing that they will encounter surgeons who choose not to use the hands-free technique, and we want them to be safe in this practice as well.

Learners often have difficulty determining the difference between the Crile, mosquito, Pean, and Kelly forceps. The textbooks label them as forceps. In the practice setting, they are commonly called clamps because they are used for clamping and occluding tissue. In an effort to assist learners to resolve this initial confusion, we introduce the clamps at the same time as the forceps, ask them to compare the length of the instrument and the sharpness or bluntness of the tips, and then describe the tissues and procedures for which each clamp is used. We look at the clamps on the stringer and discuss how they are encountered in the counting process. Also, in the initial study of basic instruments, learners often confuse the Allis, Babcock, and Kocher. These forceps (clamps) are in the grasping-and-holding category. We contrast and compare these clamps (traumatic and atraumatic) and describe their use in the surgical setting. Because Alice (Allis) is a woman's name, we use that analogy but, of course, in contemporary American society this is not a common female name. As learners progress through their studies, a test question might ask them to list the instruments they would place on their Mayo stand for a particular procedure. Again, we emphasize on which instrument trays these clamps are commonly used.

At first appearance, laparoscopy instruments seem complex to the novice. Demonstrating these instruments and explaining that they serve the same function and often have the same or similar names only on a longer, different type of handle, helps to ease the learner's anxiety.

Today's learners are comfortable finding information on the Internet to assist them in acquiring knowledge about surgical instruments. There are many sites that we guide learners to. These include:

- Instrument manufacturer's sites—online catalogs, downloads
- Content on surgical instruments or surgical instrument images found using a search engine
- Flash card exchanges
- Videos of surgical instruments in use
- Podcast prepared by instructor.

Introducing surgical instrumentation to the novice is challenging and rewarding. A great sense of pride and accomplishment is evident when new perioperative nurses, surgical technologists, or nursing students complete their first instrument counts smoothly and efficiently; when novices are scrubbed for a procedure and they anticipate the needs of the surgeon with the appropriate instrument based on their knowledge of the procedure and the instrumentation; and the first time novice nurses or technologists recognize that an instrument is not functioning correctly and remove it from service. By these learning outcomes, the instructor or preceptor recognizes that the learners are on their way to providing safe, high quality patient care. There are always new procedures and new instruments being developed. The learning never ends; it is a career-long process.

REFERENCES

1. Oermann MH, Gaberson KB. Assessment and the educational process. In: Evaluation and testing in nursing education. 3rd edition. New York: Springer Publishing; 2009. p. 16–25.
2. Bloom BS, Englehart MD, Furst EJ, et al. Taxonomy of educational objectives: the classification of educational goals. Handbook I: cognitive domain. White Plains (NY): Longman; 1956.
3. Krathwohl D, Bloom B, Masia B. Taxonomy of educational objectives. Handbook II: affective domain. New York: Longman; 1964.
4. Dave RH. Psychomotor levels. In: Armstrong RJ, editor. Developing and writing behavioral objectives. Tucson (AZ): Educational Innovators; 1970.

Surgical Instruments: A Laughing Matter?

Stephanie Smith Stanfield, RN, BSN, CNOR

KEYWORDS

- Surgical instruments • Humor • Jokes
- Perioperative nursing

Humor can serve many purposes in the operating room. It has been said that we rarely tease someone we don't like. Frequently we use humor to reinforce the bonds among coworkers. Humor may be used as a teaching tool with anxious patients or new staff members. It may be used to illustrate a point to a physician or to other members of the surgical team. We also use humor to defuse tension. The members of the surgical team are under pressure at all times. There is pressure to make sure all the equipment and supplies are available for any possible permutation of each case, to prevent errors, to start on time, to turn each room over quickly, and to coexist peaceably with those who are, frankly, at times unlovable. Humor can be a way to release some of that pressure in the perioperative environment.

Among the sources of humor in the operating room (OR) are jokes or funny stories about the names or functions of surgical instruments or equipment. This article presents a collection of such jokes and stories, arranged in various categories, contributed by perioperative nurses and other members of the surgical team.

The first category comprises jokes or pranks used to tease or poke fun at new staff members or students. This type of humor is a form of hazing, and it can be hurtful if the novice takes offense at being the object of the prank. But it is a common way to "initiate" new members of the surgical team. If the joke does not result in public humiliation, the new person often enjoys the good-natured teasing. Here are a couple of examples of common initiation jokes or pranks:

I'm sure you know the old one about sending the "newbie" out for an Otis elevator. It is, of course, the elevator that takes you between floors, not a surgical instrument. The manufacturer was in Toledo, Ohio, and the company was eventually bought by another elevator company, but you can still see "Otis" nameplates on some old elevators. The poor newbie would come back distraught after not being able to find the instrument and the surgeon would say something like "I don't know why you can't find one; didn't you ride it up to the operating room this morning?" (From Marrice King, RN, BSN, CNOR; Also submitted by Sheila

North Brownsville Surgery Center, 5700 North Expressway, Suite 201, Brownsville, TX 78526, USA
E-mail address: Stephanie.Stanfield@valleybaptist.net

Perioperative Nursing Clinics 5 (2010) 89–93
doi:10.1016/j.cpen.2009.12.003
1556-7931/10/$ – see front matter © 2010 Elsevier Inc. All rights reserved.

L. Allen, RN, BSN, CNOR, CRNFA[E]; Rebecca Blades RN, BSN, CNOR, CRNFA; and Jerry S. Effner, RN)

Have you ever sent new staff members or students out of the operating room for a Henway? When they ask, "What's a Henway?," you answer, "About 6 or 7 pounds." (Henway = hen weigh—get it?) (From Kathleen B. Gaberson, PhD, RN, CNOR, CNE, ANEF)

One of the first assistants I worked with would catch new staff or students and tell them in a very offhand, conversational tone that "We're gonna need a cowsay for this next case." They would give him a blank look and sometimes say "Huh?" before the light began to dawn. Although on a couple of occasions, I did hear the question, "What's a cowsay?" and the big chuckle preceding the inevitable answer, "Moo." (From Stephanie Stanfield, RN, BSN, CNOR)

I observed an obstetrician/gynecologist famous for terrorizing new staff members send one of our student nurses to bring another weighted vaginal speculum, but he wanted a left-handed one. Fortunately, her preceptor caught her on the way out the door to let her know that there was no such thing. (From Stephanie Stanfield, RN, BSN, CNOR)

I was putting up instruments in our instrument room the other day. One of our sets was labeled "Miner Set" instead of "Minor Set"—made me smile. This is always good for a day in the OR. (From Georgia Walz, RN, CNOR)

Another category of jokes usually is created inadvertently: formulating new, informal, names for instruments, sets, or equipment, or referring to them by their "nicknames," well known by experienced surgeons and staff members. However, novices often are stymied by these names, which don't match the ones they studied so conscientiously. Sometimes the correct name is used, but novices misinterpret what they hear, and the results can be a source of humor for all observers, if not the novice.

For example, we teach nursing and surgical technologist students and new nursing staff members who are learning the scrub role how to arrange instruments on the Mayo stand while setting up a case. Maybe it's the effect of trying to talk through a surgical mask, or maybe it's due to regional accents, but sometimes we don't make ourselves clear to the poor novice, as the following example illustrates:

During the surgery rotation in nursing school, the instructor was talking about the Mayo stand. One of my fellow students finally asked, "Well, if that is the male stand, what do we use for women?" The whole class laughed for 30 minutes. I graduated in 1982 and I still fondly remember this story when teaching students and new perioperative nurses. (From Kristy Snyder, RN, BSN, CNOR)

I have some memories about names for instruments from a place where I used to work. At first I thought that the names they were using were the real names for these instruments! I was newly returning to the OR after a child-raising absence, and laparoscopic cholecystectomy were new to me. Alas, I learned that the real names were different, but I still remember what and why they were called by the other names. Now, can I remember what the real names of those instruments are? (1) "Goat grabber": This instrument is in the laparoscopic cholecystectomy set; the first time the surgeon saw it he thought it was big enough to "grab a goat." In the catalog this is listed as a claw forceps. (2) "The Sharon Stone": Another surgeon wanted the stone forceps and could never call it by the right name. Sharon Stone, the actress, was popular at the time, so he would ask for the "What's the name? Sharon something instrument." Some 10-plus years later I still smile when these instruments are used, and these docs don't know why I am smiling. (From Karen G. Hausteen, RN, CNOR)

I traveled a little bit in my OR career. At one time I worked in a hospital that did a lot of laparoscopic gastric bypass surgeries. They were kind enough to put me in sterile stores for a day putting away sterilized instruments and sets so I could find what I needed when it was needed. I was accustomed to seeing laparoscopic sets of a couple different varieties, but this facility called them all "pelviscopy sets." Not that there's anything at all amusing about that. In fact, it makes perfect sense when you think about it. The humor came as I tried for 8 weeks to pronounce it! I could parrot it back when someone else said it but to look at the label and pronounce it was just beyond me! It still tickles me when I think about that set! Another time, I was working in a small rural hospital. We had the opportunity to scrub occasionally and I always volunteered for that. One day I was assisting a surgeon who had trained somewhere else. He asked for a "snap, please" and so the tech did just that, snapping her fingers rather quietly. I thought our tech must have had other things on her mind, so I let it pass the first time and handed him a hemostat. The next time he asked for a "snap, please" and it happened again, I could barely contain my laughter. The next time he asked for a snap, I quickly put my hand over hers and handed him a hemostat. So as not to embarrass her, I took her aside after the case and explained. She laughed at herself and told me she "just couldn't figure out what he wanted" with that request, "but he must have a good reason." I never hear "snap, please" that I don't remember that tech. (From Stephanie Stanfield, RN, BSN, CNOR)

I worked with a plastic surgeon, a wonderful human being and a very capable surgeon. He was very active in teaching and mentoring. He had probably the best sterile technique I've ever witnessed. One day, (after I had formed this opinion) he asked for a "pizza board." I was shocked that this paragon of the OR would ever consider bringing in nonregulation equipment to our sterile environment. It turns out that he was asking for a board that slides under the patient's shoulders to allow application of the dressings following breast surgery. Boy, did I feel silly! (From Stephanie Stanfield, RN, BSN, CNOR)

Our colleagues on the surgical team, although not novices, may also be affected by this type of verbal shorthand. I received this story from a certified registered nurse anesthetist:

My first day providing anesthesia in a plastic surgery office proved to be interesting. During a liposuction, the surgeon shouted, "Step on the roach!" I immediately began looking around on the floor, thinking, "Holy crap, they have roaches running around here!" No one else in the room seemed to be bothered by this situation. Then I looked over to find the circulator stepping on the small round foot pedal to activate the liposuction equipment!! I continued to be nonchalant while laughing hysterically inside at myself for thinking there would be live roaches in the OR!! That was 6 months ago and I still chuckle when I hear that said. (From Kim Russell, CRNA)

This event took place many years ago when I was a very "green" nursing student in a diploma school of nursing. My OR rotation was the first one after the 6-month probationary period, and I was terrified because there were so many unfamiliar things to learn and every staff member seemed to expect nursing students to know as much as they did. I was especially terrified of the licensed practical nurses and surgical technologists who performed the scrub role in many of the surgical services. One scrub person in particular made my stomach churn and my knees turn to jelly every time she spoke to me. She was the regular scrub person on the plastic surgery service. Of course, because nursing students rotated among all services, one day it was my turn to work with her. Before she started to scrub, she told me to go to the sterile core and see if the plastic instruments were ready. So off I went, and because no one was there to ask, I just looked around and I didn't see any plastic instruments at all. In fact, they were all stainless steel. The scrub person was not happy when I reported this information back to her. (From Kathleen B. Gaberson, PhD, RN, CNOR, CNE, ANEF)

The final category of surgical instrument jokes involves the challenge of communicating with others on the surgical team when tension levels are high. Who among us hasn't forgotten the name of a person or object when we are stressed, distracted, angry, or fatigued? After all, that's why hand signals were developed for the surgeon or first assistant to wordlessly communicate the need for an instrument that does "this" (cut, grasp, retract) without taking his or her focus from the incision. Well, what happens when a surgeon can't remember the name of the specific instrument he wants and the scrub person is so new that he or she can't anticipate that need? This final story took place decades ago when the writer was a nursing student and when verbal abuse of OR nurses by surgeons was much more common. This would probably never happen today (or would it?).

I was a young nursing student in my OR rotation. I was getting fairly comfortable with general surgery cases, but up to this point, I had always been second scrub or I was first scrub on a very simple case with an experienced person as second scrub to guide me. One day, I was scheduled to second scrub for Dr X. He was known for having quite a temper and for using crude language. The first scrub was a young registered nurse, let's call her Susan, who was obviously pregnant. As the case started, Dr X began to make remarks about Susan's fecund state. She ignored him at first. Then he began to ask questions in a joking manner about the sexual activities that had resulted in that pregnancy. She put the instrument she was about to pass to him on the Mayo stand, and calmly but firmly said, "Dr X, if you make one more personal remark about me, I will leave this case." He was quiet for a few minutes, but soon started up again with a teasing comment about her pregnancy. Susan said, "That's it. I'm leaving." And she stepped back from the sterile field, removed her gloves and gown, and left the room. Dr X threw one instrument after her, which hit the wall and then the floor. I was standing at the back table, stunned and unmoving, until the circulator whispered, "Get up there!" As I was repositioning myself at the Mayo stand, Dr X angrily shouted, "Give me....give me a....you know...." while making hand motions that I could not interpret. I started holding up instruments that were on the Mayo stand. Kelly? No? Scissors? No? Help me out a little bit here! Give me a hint! I hoped against hope that what he was asking for wasn't the instrument that he had thrown, but soon it became apparent that he wanted something on the back table. So I turned slightly to look at the large number of instruments available there. By that time I had forgotten where we were in the case, so I couldn't even anticipate the general category of instruments that he needed next. So I turned back to look at him and said, "What do you want?" In anger and frustration, he sputtered, "Give me one of those...those...silver things!" The room was dead silent as I replied, "Dr X, I have a whole back table full of silver things. You're going to have to be more specific than that." Still lost for the name of the instrument he wanted, Dr X proceeded to mimic with hand motions the movement of a coiled snake. That's when I finally realized that he wanted a cobra retractor, and I located it and passed it to him. He never said another word the rest of the case. I vowed never to work in the OR after I graduated. Good thing I didn't keep that vow! (From Kathleen B. Gaberson, PhD, RN, CNOR, CNE)

Although each of these stories is unique to the specific time and place in which it happened, every perioperative nurse can appreciate the inherent humor. These stories have demonstrated the power of humor to release tension, relieve boredom, convey comradeship, compensate for memory lapse, stimulate creativity, and make a demanding job enjoyable, if only for a moment. Shared laughter is a way to help members of the surgical team connect and communicate. Whether intentional or unintentional, humor is an integral element of perioperative nursing.[1]

Thank you to all perioperative nurses and colleagues who contributed to this collection of surgical instrument jokes. They demonstrate in many ways that sometimes surgical instrumentation *is* a laughing matter!

REFERENCE

1. Tunistra SEB. You had to be there: true stories of humor in the OR. Semin Perioper Nurs 1999;8(2):88–94.

Index

Note: Page numbers of article titles are in **bold face** type.

A

Aesop robot, 69–70
Affective domain, teaching instrumentation techniques and, 84–85
Anesthesia, history of, 6–7
Antisepsis and asepsis, history of, 7–9
Assistive technology, for instrument count, 39
Australian Safety and Efficacy Register of New Interventional Procedures, 63
Availability, of instrumentation, 21

B

Behavior, disruptive, instrument errors related to, 22–23
Blood-borne injuries, reduction of
    hands-free technique for, **45–58,** 63
    scalpel safety in, **59–67**

C

Cardiac surgery, robotic, 79
Cesarean births, hands-free technique use during, 48–49
Cleaning, of robotic instruments, 80
Cognitive domain, teaching instrumentation techniques and, 84
Console, of robots, 72–73
Counts, instrument, evidence-supported best practices for, **27–44**
    assistive technology for, 39
    counting process, 32–39
    implementation of, 39, 41–42
    literature search on, 28–29
    new paradigm for, 27–28
    protocols for, 29
    recommendations for, 39
    retained object events, 28, 30–32
    terminology for, 38

D

daVinci Surgical System, 70–74, 78, 80
Disinfection, of robotic instruments, 80
Disposable instrumentation, 11
Distraction, instrument errors related to, 23
Draping, for robotic surgery, 75–76

Perioperative Nursing Clinics 5 (2010) 95–99
doi:10.1016/S1556-7931(10)00002-1
1556-7931/10/$ – see front matter © 2010 Elsevier Inc. All rights reserved.
periopnursing.theclinics.com

E

Efficiency programs, 23–24
EndoWrist instrument, 70, 77
Engineered sharps injury prevention devices, 61–62

F

Fatigue, instrument errors related to, 23

G

Galen, 3
Glove tears, reduction of, hands-free technique for, **45–58,** 63
Gynecologic surgery, robotic, 79–80
Gyrus robot, 78–79

H

Hands-free technique, **45–58**
    clinical studies on, 48–54
    description of, 46–48
    for scalpel handling, 63
    increasing use of, 54–55
    rates of, 54
Hermes robot, 70
Hippocrates, 2–3
History. *See* Instrumentation, history of.
Humor, related to instrumentation, **89–93**

I

Information resources, for instrument techniques, 85–87
Institute for Clinical System Improvement, surgical count protocol of, 29
Institute of Medicine, safety report of, 18
Instrumentation
    counting of, **27–44**
    for robotic surgery, **69–81**
    hands-free technique for, **45–58,** 63
    history of, **1–13,** 3–4
        ancient, 2–3
        anesthesia introduction, 6–7
        antisepsis and asepsis, 7–9
        Middle Ages, 3–5
        modern era, 9–11
        Renaissance, 5–6
        war surgery, 4–5, 7–11
    humor related to, **89–93**
    readiness of, **15–25**
    scalpel safety in, **59–67**
    teaching of, **83–88**
Interruptions, instrument errors related to, 23

J

Jokes, related to instrumentation, **89–93**

L

Learning, domains of, 83–85
Legislation, for sharps injury prevention, 61
Lister, Joseph, 8
Lithotomy, in Middle Ages, 4

N

National Patient Safety Goals, 19
National Quality Forum's Severe Reportable Events list, 27
Needle injuries, reduction of, hands-free technique for, **45–58,** 63
Needlestick Safety and Prevention Act, 61
Nightingale, Florence, 7

P

Paré (surgeon), 5
Pasteur, Louis, 8
Pranks, related to instrumentation, **89–93**
Psychomotor domain, teaching instrumentation techniques and, 85

R

Readiness, instrument, **15–25**
    availability in, 21
    definition of, 16–18
    for efficiency, 23–24
    lack of
        distraction-induced, 23
        fatigue-related, 23
        interruptions and, 23
        scenarios for, 15–16
        stress-related, 22–23
        substitutions for, 21–22
    safety and, 18–21
Regulations, on scalpel safety, 63–65
Retained object events, 28, 30–32
"Review of Patient Safety in the Operating Room in Veterans Health Administration
    Facilities," 17, 21
Robotic surgery systems, **69–81**
    advantages of, 60
    cleaning of, 80
    components of, 71–74
    disadvantages of, 60–61
    disinfection of, 80
    draping for, 75–76

Robotic (*continued*)
    economic issues with, 80
    handling components of, 75
    history of, 69–70
    instrumentation for, 76–79
    maintenance of, 75
    shut-down procedure for, 79–80

S

Safety
    hands-free technique for, **45–58**, 63
    in scalpel handling, **59–67**
    instrument counts for, **27–44**
    instrument readiness for, **15–25**
Scalpel safety, **59–67**
    devices for, 61–62
    financial aspects of, 60
    human implications of, 60
    importance of, 60
    infection risk and, 59–60
    legislation on, 61
    new paradigm for, 63
    regulations on, 63–65
    safety scalpels for, 62–63
Second Global Patient Safety Challenge: Safe Surgery Saves Lives, 19
Semmelweis, Ignnaz, 7
Sentinel Event Alerts, 18–19
Service Employees International Union, on sharps injury prevention legislation, 61
Severe Reportable Events list, 27
Sharps injuries
    financial consequences of, 60
    human costs of, 60
    preventive devices for, 61–62
    reduction of
        hands-free technique for, **45–58**, 63
        scalpel safety in, **59–67**
Socrates robot, 70
"Standards for Sponge, Needle, and Instrument Procedures," 28
Sterilization, of robotic instruments, 80
Stress, instrument errors related to, 22–23
Substitutions, for instruments, 21–22
Surgical Safety Checklist, 19–21

T

Teaching, of surgical instrumentation, **83–88**
    domains of learning and, 83–85
    effective approaches to, 85–88
Textbooks, for instrument techniques, 85–87
Throughput, promotion of, 23–24

"To Err is Human: Building a Safer Health System," 18
Trephination, ancient tools for, 2

U

Universal Precautions, 19, 61
Urologic surgery, robotic, 79–80

V

Versalius, 4–5
Veterans Health Administration, surgical count protocol of, 29
Vision system, for robots, 71

W

War surgery
    in ancient times, 3
    in 1800s, 7–8
    in Middle Ages, 4–5
    in 1900s, 9–11
World Alliance for Patient Safety, 19
World Health Organization
    surgical count protocol of, 29
    surgical safety initiatives of, 19–21

Z

Zeus Robotic Surgical System, 70

Moving?

Make sure your subscription moves with you!

To notify us of your new address, find your **Clinics Account Number** (located on your mailing label above your name), and contact customer service at:

Email: journalscustomerservice-usa@elsevier.com

800-654-2452 (subscribers in the U.S. & Canada)
314-447-8871 (subscribers outside of the U.S. & Canada)

Fax number: 314-447-8029

Elsevier Health Sciences Division
Subscription Customer Service
3251 Riverport Lane
Maryland Heights, MO 63043

*To ensure uninterrupted delivery of your subscription, please notify us at least 4 weeks in advance of move.

Printed and bound by CPI Group (UK) Ltd, Croydon, CR0 4YY

03/10/2024

01040462-0011